Tse-loh-ne
(The People at the End of the Rocks)

TSE-LOH-NE
(The People at the End of the Rocks)

Journey Down the Davie Trail

Keith Billington

CAITLIN PRESS

Copyright © 2012 Keith Billington

01 02 03 04 05 06 17 16 15 14 13 12

All rights reserved. No part of this publication may be reproduced, stored in a retrieval system or transmitted, in any form or by any means, without prior permission of the publisher or, in the case of photocopying or other reprographic copying, a licence from Access Copyright, the Canadian Copyright Licensing Agency, www.accesscopyright.ca, 1-800-893-5777, info@accesscopyright.ca.

Caitlin Press Inc.
8100 Alderwood Road,
Halfmoon Bay, BC V0N 1Y1
www.caitlin-press.com

Text design by Kathleen Fraser.
Cover design by Vici Johnstone.
Edited by Catherine Edwards.
Printed in Canada.

Caitlin Press Inc. acknowledges financial support from the Government of Canada through the Canada Book Fund and the Canada Council for the Arts, and from the Province of British Columbia through the British Columbia Arts Council and the Book Publisher's Tax Credit.

Library and Archives Canada Cataloguing in Publication
Billington, Keith, 1940-
    Tse-loh-ne (the people at the end of the rocks) : journey down the Davie Trail / Keith Billington.

ISBN 978-1-894759-88-5

    1. Billington, Keith, 1940-. 2. Sekani Indians—Social life and customs. 3. Sekani Indians—Social conditions. 4. Male nurses—British Columbia—Fort Ware—Biography. I. Title.

RT37.B54A3 2012   610.73092   C2012-903333-2

This book is dedicated to all the elders of Fort Ware who have walked hundreds of miles on trails throughout their homeland. Special thanks go to Charlie and Hazel Boya, Tommy Poole and Chief Emil McCook who shared so many travels and stories with me.

Principal Andreas Rohrbach and the Aatse Davie Education Committee allowed me to copy some of their photographs as did Dennis at W.D. West photographers in Prince George.

Catherine Edwards of UBC has been invaluable for her editorial skills. Thanks to Jay Sherwood for his support and advice.

I could not have written this book without the encouragement and support of my wife, Muriel, who was always there at the end of the trail.

Keith Billington
Prince George, BC

Contents

Introduction	11
Prologue	13
In the Beginning…	15
Trails to Ware	18
Just a Matter of Time	21
Flying by the Seat of My Pants	25
Listen to the Band	30
The People at the End of the Rocks	35
Take a Walk	42
Charlie Boya	46
The Store	51
The Accident	56
Serengeti of the North	60
The Road, the Lake, and the Booze	66
Circuit Court	70
Mapping the Davie Trail	77
These Boots Are Made for Walking	86
Watch Out for Bear!	90
That's Life on the Trail!	96
Too Little, Too Much Water	110
Crossing the Red River	116
Bad Memories	120
Plane Crash Survivors	124
Scoop Lake	127
John Ogilvie "Skookum" Davidson	138
The Turnagain River	146
Things Old and Things New	151
A Grizzly Surprise	160
A Grave Concern	164

Gataga Forks	168
The Crossing	175
City Cabin	182
Boot Hill	187
Lone Creek to Rudolph's Cut Bank	193
Helicopter Evacuation	202
Hunger and Thirst	210
Baby Lakes	219
Fox Lake	226
Beaver Pass and the Bedaux Sub-Arctic Expedition	237
Old Friends and Home	243
Epilogue	250
Further Reading	252

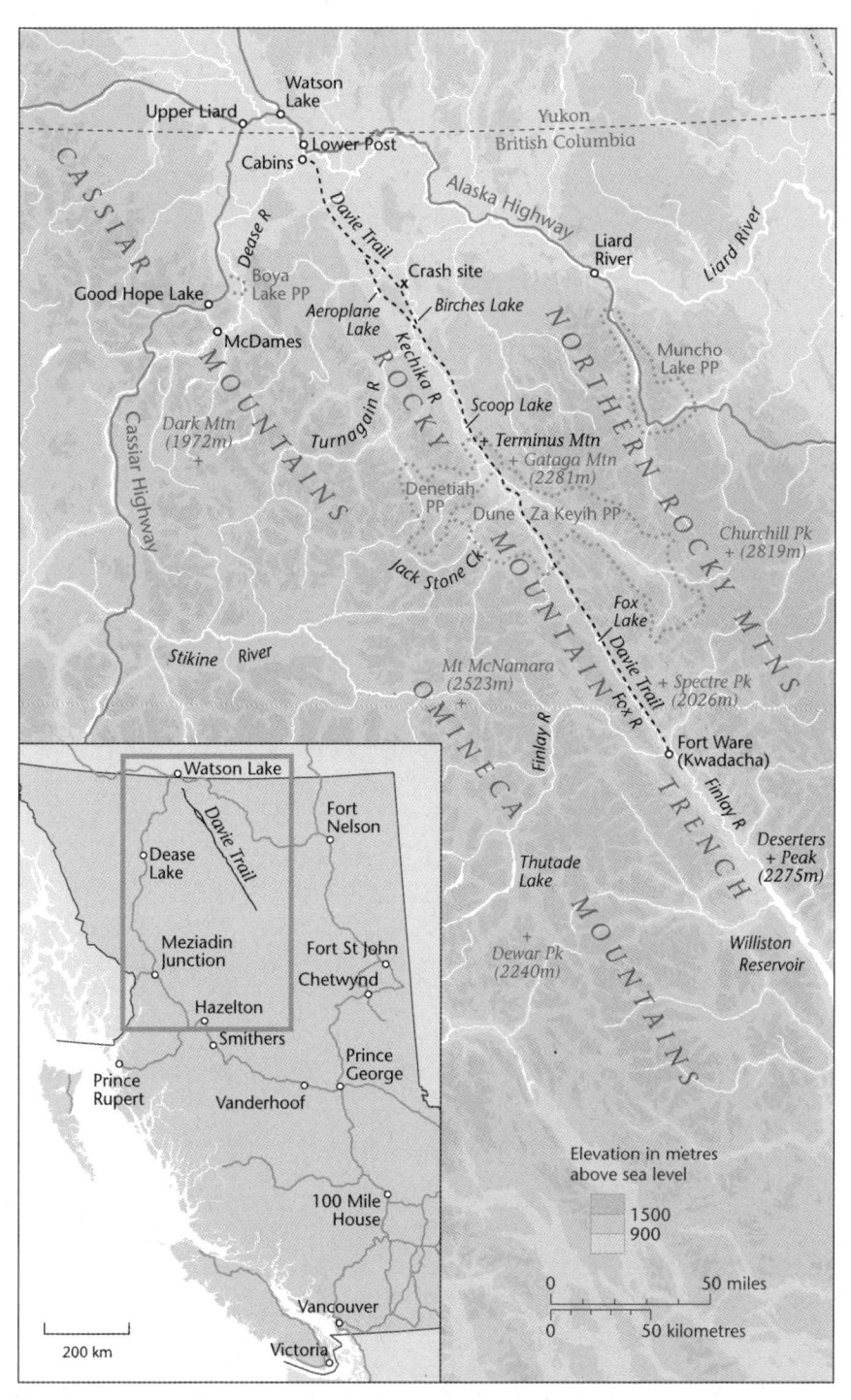

Map by Eric Leinberger.

Introduction

In 1969, Keith Billington and his wife, Muriel, moved to British Columbia from the Northwest Territories, where they had worked as outpost nurses. *House Calls by Dogsled* (Harbour, 2008) and *Cold Land, Warm Hearts* (Harbour, 2010) record memoirs of their life and experiences there. In British Columbia, Keith continued working with and for the First Nations of the northern Interior, first working for the Federal Health Services providing remote health care, then later working for the Sekani Band in Fort Ware as the Band Manager.

Keith began working as the Band Manager for the Sekani Band in 1988, at the request of the Fort Ware Chief and Council. Along with his new responsibilities, he found that his past experience and skills were frequently called upon: he did dental work, sutured wounds, delivered babies that couldn't wait, acted as an ambulance driver and prepared deceased persons for burial.

The People at the End of the Rocks describes the lifestyle and history of the Kaska and Sekani people who live in the most isolated village in British Columbia. Through Keith's many adventures, the reader has a glimpse into the hardships and rigours experienced by a people who have one foot in their past and the other foot in the future as they try to adapt to today's values with some reluctance, knowing that change is inevitable.

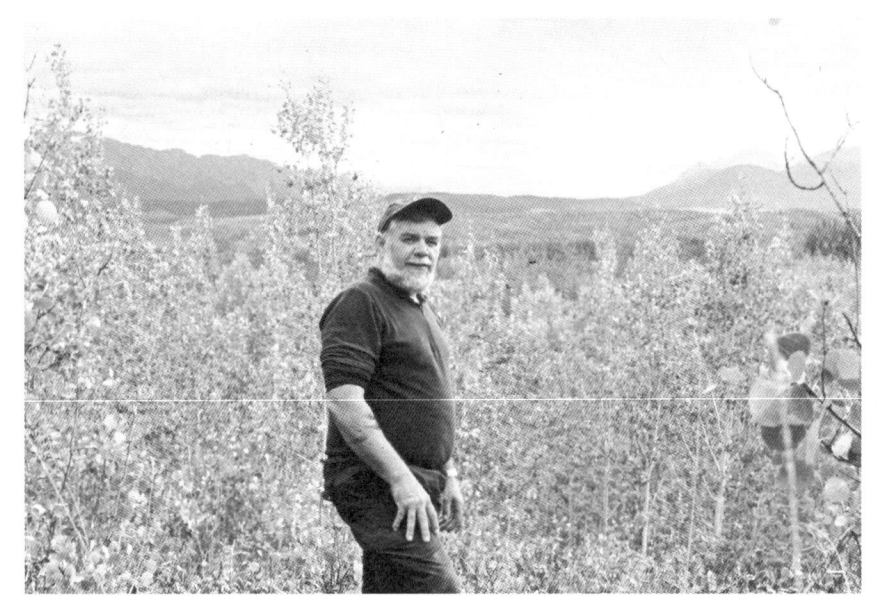

Only 460 kilometres to go, eh? Author Keith Billington on the Aatse Davie Trail.

During a 460-kilometre hike through Kaska and Sekani territory on the Aatse Davie Trail, Keith blends some of the joys and tribulations with stories of the realities of the Sekani life. *The People at the End of the Rocks* brings together events that have occurred in the past in this wilderness area, which is still on the very frontier of British Columbia, but is now in danger of changing radically as its resources come into demand.

Prologue

A birthday present that almost guarantees that you will lose twenty pounds would delight most people and I was excited to receive such an invitation. The downside of the invitation was the seventy-pound pack I was going to have to carry for 460 kilometres along a little-known trail in the Rocky Mountain Trench.

I had been the Band Manager for the Fort Ware Indian Band for over ten years, and had travelled on the Finlay River by river boat and over many of the local trails by snowshoe, snowmobile, and on skis, but the trail that fascinated me most was the Aatse Davie Trail that ran from Lower Post on the northern border of British Columbia to Fort Ware in north-central BC.

Charlie and Hazel Boya were the only people who were familiar with the trail, having both spent part of their childhoods on the trail and having walked it many times over the years. Now they were talking about hiking the trail again to ensure that it would be part of the Band's land claims strategy when the Band, a member of the Kaska Tribal Council, entered into negotiations with the government.

"We have a birthday present for you, Keith," Charlie announced one evening when I was visiting him and his wife, Hazel. Charlie and I had been friends for years and I spent a lot of time at the Boyas' house drinking coffee and listening to the tales Charlie told. Charlie knew that I had a great desire to walk the Davie Trail, having heard so much about it from him.

"What's it going to cost me?" I asked, knowing that Charlie always had a scheme going that would cost me money.

"How would you like to walk down the Davie Trail with us and really experience how we used to live in the bush?"

I was delighted and excited at the prospect. I knew that the Kaska were doing everything they could to document their relationship to their land, and that they had negotiated with an environmental group in Williams Lake for Eric Gunderson to do some mapping for them. At the time I didn't mention that my upcoming birthday was going to be my sixtieth—it was going to be now or never!

"When shall I start packing?"

In the Beginning…

The Jet Ranger helicopter flew north for two hours along Williston Lake and then up the Finlay River. After sighting a small cabin, the pilot brought the machine down from three thousand feet, banked to the right, and descended with the nose tilted slightly up to a landing on the riverbank. The downdraft from the huge rotors whisked leaves and debris into the fast-flowing river. A few dogs tied up behind the cabin took refuge in their broken-down boxes and then, as the noise and motion slowed down, a man peered out of the cabin door and walked slowly towards us.

He was a tall, lean, angular man dressed in blue jeans and a black western shirt. His shoulder-length black hair was crowned with a black cowboy hat. He smiled and walked over and greeted me, shaking my hand in the brief handshake used by most First Nations people. He told me that his name was Emil McCook and that he was the Chief of the Fort Ware Indian Band.

After exchanging a few words of greeting, I explained why I had literally dropped in at his cabin in a helicopter and asked if I could take a sample of blood and cut a small swatch of hair from each member of his family. I was employed at that time by "Indian Health"—part of the federal department of Health and Welfare. I travelled throughout northern BC as a nurse working on special projects. This one required me to collect blood and hair samples

16   Tse-loh-ne

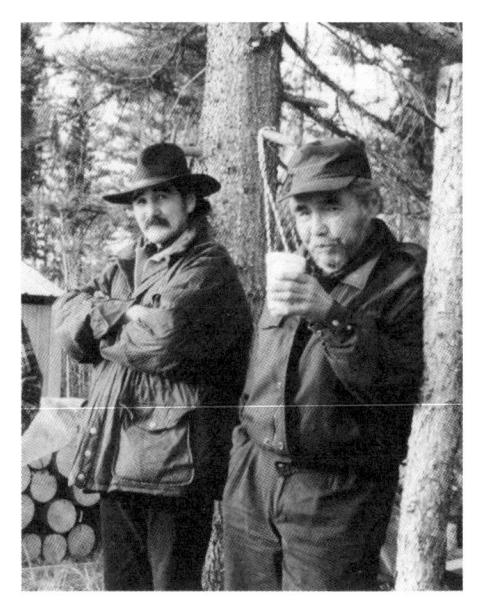

Chief Emil McCook and Councillor Tommy Poole.

from First Nations men, women, children and babies and to have it tested for mercury poisoning.

In 1960, Minamata disease, or mercury poisoning caused by industrial pollution, was discovered. It was caused by people eating fish contaminated with methyl mercury from polluted rivers and seas near Minamata, Japan. Concern emerged that Aboriginal peoples with a diet containing substantial amounts of fish—and who also lived near mine sites, as the Fort Ware Band did—might also develop this disease, and the tests I conducted grew out of this concern.

The Chief was very cooperative and asked me to follow him into his small cabin. It was built of unpeeled logs on the bank of the Finlay River, with Prairie Mountain rising steeply behind it. Small children ran around and stared with awe at the helicopter and then ran and hid as I made my way over to the cabin with Emil. The dogs tied up behind the cabin now greeted us with loud barks and Emil gave them a curt shout, which silenced them. A small pocket-sized dog ran around loose, looking quite out of place in this environment. Later, I found out that this little creature was the special pet of Fanny McCook, the Chief's wife.

Considering that I had arrived unannounced, the Chief seemed to accept my presence as quite an ordinary event. I found out later that Emil had been dealing with government bureaucrats both in Fort Ware and down south for many years and nothing I did was likely to surprise him.

The cabin was hot, with a woodstove burning even though it was a warm day. When Fanny McCook asked if I would like tea, I realized the stove was necessary for cooking. The Chief's wife was a large woman and looked a bit severe, but she was quite shy and I found that she covered her shyness by being quiet as she went about her business. Later, I was to see that she had a great sense of humour and loved to tease.

Several small children giggled and peeked shyly out of a small bedroom, jostling one another so that they could get a better look at this bearded stranger who had suddenly descended upon them. When I repeated my request after telling Fanny why I was there, she called out in a loud voice, "You kids come here!" They crowded into the main room of the cabin, giggling, and tried to hide behind Fanny, peering at me from the safety of their mother.

I took samples of hair and blood from Emil and Fanny, then Fanny called the children forward. So far they had thought that it was a lot of fun as their parents submitted to my probes. They came forward willingly enough to have their hair samples cut—but when they realized that the syringe and needle I was preparing was for one of them and I started to take a blood sample, they suddenly became reluctant and the older children pushed the smaller ones in front of them. As each patient had a Band-Aid applied, the next one asked in a small voice, "Does it hurt?" Finally, with Fanny's help, I completed my task and told Emil that I would send him the test results when they had been processed. (Fortunately, the test results didn't indicate any problems.)

Emil had a long river boat tied up on the Finlay River, a boat he had built himself, he told me proudly when I asked him about it. Going with the river current, he could travel down to Fort Ware in about half an hour, although it took him longer coming back, especially if the boat was loaded.

I chatted with the Chief and his wife for a while and asked about any other people living in the area. They told me that most people would be in the village at this time because it was the start of the school year. His children, who could now see that all danger to their bodies was over, escorted us to the helicopter with shouts and giggles, demonstrating their relief as we prepared to depart.

As the helicopter took off, the family was soon engulfed by the trees, the river and the mountains. As I looked down at them waving at us, we swept over towards the village. I had no idea then how the future would bring me into a close relationship with them all.

Trails to Ware

When I moved to Prince George in 1973 and was getting to know where the various Indian Reserves were, I had flown north in a small blue and white Cessna 185 airplane operated by Northern Thunderbird Air. As the pilot flew north up the Rocky Mountain Trench over the forests and lakes of this northeastern section of British Columbia, I could see far below me a few small cabins scattered here and there by the side of winding rivers and turquoise blue lakes. Snowcapped mountains running in a northwesterly direction served as a backdrop to this very Canadian scene.

My eye was caught by bright orange and blue tarpaulins below us that covered caches of food and supplies, looking out of place amongst the greens and browns of the surrounding country. It seemed incredible that people lived down there amongst the rivers, trees and majestic mountains, walking the trails I could see snaking through the trees in every direction, and probably taking weeks to make the same journey that the plane was now making in hours. I thought about how these people would have to be physically fit men, women and children who accepted the hard work of surviving in the elements as part of everyday life. From my vantage point in the air, the most prominent trail, heading north, followed the winding, serpentine Finlay River—later I learned that this was the Davie Trail.

The view from the plane that day aroused my curiosity about the people who lived in this very remote area of northern British Columbia and I looked forward to talking with them and learning more about their way of life. I had long been intrigued by what I had read about the lifestyle of the people in this remote area and from what I had heard, I was reminded of the Gwich'in people of Fort McPherson in the Northwest Territories where my wife and I had lived for six years. All I knew at the time, though, was that the people far below the airplane were Sekani people and that their village, Fort Ware, had been named years ago when the Hudson's Bay Company had built a trading post there at the confluence of the Kwadacha, Finlay and Fox rivers.

The Finlay River flows from the west. Its headwaters originate in Thutade Lake (pronounced "Toodaddy"), which means "long, narrow lake" in the Sekani language, located in the North Swannell Range, close to where the giant Kemess mine now operates. Fort Ware is situated on a triangular piece of land between the Fox River to the north, the Kwadacha to the east, and the Finlay to the west.

I wondered how these First Nations people survived. Isolated from the south long before the dam that created Williston Lake was constructed by BC Hydro in the late 1960s, Fort Ware was separated from the rest of British Columbia by its location far from any roads to the north, south, east or west. After the largest earth-filled dam in North America had been built at Hudson's Hope in the Peace River Canyon, thousands of hectares of the Rocky Mountain Trench were flooded, becoming Williston Lake, and effectively cutting off the vital river boat access to Fort Ware from the Crooked, Parsnip and lower Finlay rivers that were south of the village. An already isolated community had become even more isolated. Village supplies and government services now had to be flown in by small float or ski-equipped aircraft, which is why I was now flying in to the village.

When I worked in the Northwest Territories in an equally isolated village, I was painfully aware of the difficulties experienced by the First Nations people who either paid high prices for or went without the supplies that everyone else in the country takes for granted. It was good to know that in the far north, roads and improved communications had now changed the people's lives to a great extent. This part of British Columbia, however, was still fifty years or more behind everyone else.

An old Gwich'in man in the Northwest Territories had told me that the white people who came to his village could never really understand what it was like to live in their country unless they travelled through it like they did, without all the comforts that usually surround visitors. I suspected that most of the Sekani people in this northern part of the province would share those sentiments, and I determined that, with the help of the Sekani people, I would find out what it was like to walk these trails and experience the way of life of the old-timers who spent their lives surviving in this harsh environment.

Just a Matter of Time

Because there was a critical shortage of nurses, I had the opportunity to make several more visits to Fort Ware to hold clinics. When I became the Nursing Supervisor of Community Health Nurses in northeastern British Columbia, I found that, as is the case in many supervisory jobs, there was a lot more paperwork than I liked to do. Flying to Fort Ware was an opportunity that I looked forward to—a nice change from the office grind.

On one occasion, after a two-hour plane ride from Prince George, I could see the winding Finlay River below, its clear waters washing around willow-covered gravel bars and around steep white mud cliffs. A small cluster of houses situated along the riverbank—the village of Fort Ware—came into view and the pilot circled the village after radioing his approach to Fort Nelson aeradio. I saw small figures running towards the river in expectation of seeing something or someone new. The single-engine Cessna aircraft banked sharply and the pilot approached the river from the south, dropping lower and lower until I could feel the drag of the pontoons on the water. The pilot expertly brought the plane close to the bank, keeping the engine power on to counteract the seven-knot river current. A man on shore grabbed the wing tip and the pilot cut the engine. He hastily exited the plane, grabbed a rope that was fastened to the pontoon, jumped ashore and secured the plane. After climbing down onto the pontoons and jumping ashore myself, I watched the pilot unload my supplies onto the riverbank. I walked down to the small log cabin that served as a clinic and found that the waiting room was already filling up with prospective patients. Jim Van Somer kindly picked up my equipment from the plane and delivered it to the cabin in his small Jeep.

Jim Van Somer owned and operated a small trading post in Fort Ware. He had taken over the store when his brother Art had suddenly died. Jim was quite familiar with the people of Fort Ware and was one of those hardy men who were known as the "Crooked River Rats." These "Rats" used long river boats to transport supplies from McLeod Lake to Fort Ware before Williston Lake was created, about 500 kilometres by river. It was a strenuous occupation and it took great skill to keep the boats underway without swamping the cargo. Jim—who had also been a "white trapper"—married a McLeod Lake First Nations woman, Louise. (Jim and Louise would have been very proud to see their youngest son, Donny, become the Chief of the Fort Ware Band many years later, after the children of First Nations women were accepted on the Indian Affairs Band Roll.) Jim's store was the source of groceries and also served as the post office. He had the only radio phone in the village and operated an unofficial taxi service from the plane to the clinic or the school. He was the watchman and caretaker of the clinic, and he and Louise could always be relied on to offer a cup of coffee to visitors.

I had been able to get a message to Jim about our proposed visit on his radio phone. He dutifully let people know about it when they came to his store, so I wasn't too surprised to see a full waiting room. I unpacked my bags, found the patient files and put on a pot of coffee. It was mid-morning and the plane ride had left me with a dry throat, probably from talking to the pilot too much!

As I surveyed the crowded waiting room, I couldn't help thinking about the medical and dental clinics that my wife, Muriel, and I had held at the nursing station in Fort McPherson. I could sympathize with southern doctors who had waiting rooms filled with people who, for the most part, could "take an Aspirin and call me tomorrow." As harsh as it sounds, many people suffered from aches and pains and runny noses that were part of the aging process, the result of a hard lifestyle, or simply common colds that would improve in a few days with or without medication. Over-the-counter pain relief tablets would help but there were no cures for the vagaries of life and, for the patients in Fort Ware, there were few or no over-the-counter medications available.

On the other hand, there were always a few patients who were genuinely sick and who needed medicine prescribed. Our constant worry was that an infant or young child would be moderately ill and become dehydrated or overheated in a stifling wood-heated cabin. Antibiotics were distributed reluctantly and with the firm order that the patient take the medicine until it was all gone. (So many people take their medicines only until they feel better. Then the bacteria that caused the ailment is not killed and could become resistant to the medicine.) If the antibiotic was stopped too soon, the patient could have a relapse because the bug recovered before the patient did.

One of the peculiarities of bureaucracy was that people who had medical emergencies could have their way paid to travel to Prince George for treatment, but dental patients had to either find their own way out or suffer. If a patient had a dental problem that was beyond my bush dentistry, I asked them how they felt otherwise, hoping that they could exaggerate an ache or pain so they could be referred out for tests and see a dentist while they were in town.

I was reminded of a cartoon that reflected the dilemma of people living in remote areas. Two patients were watching as a plane was landing, bringing a doctor to the village. The caption read, "Better be ill today because the doctor will be here!" This probably explained why clinics filled up with prospective patients—"just in case" they got sick when the doctor or nurse was not there.

A few years later, and much to my surprise, I received a letter from Chief Emil McCook and the Band Council. They were experiencing some administrative problems, and asked me if I would consider acting as their Band Manager. At that time, Fort Ware was described by many people as being like the Wild West of years gone by. Stories of shootings and stabbings and beatings were all thrown around by any group that had had dealings with the Fort Ware Band, and I am sure many of these stories were true. What the tale-tellers failed to mention was the alcohol, brought in to the community by bootleggers and sold for very high prices, that often fuelled these disputes and created a situation reminiscent of the eighteenth century. In spite of Fort Ware's reputation, I seriously considered this offer. After working in the Northwest Territories, I had some idea of what First Nations Bands wanted and needed and felt I could be useful, although I was ignorant of government policies and procedures regarding such programs as housing, schools, roads and finances. With the assurance that John Pateman, the Band's consulting accountant, would guide me through these things, I accepted the challenge with some trepidation and lots of excitement, not knowing what adventures awaited me.

Flying by the Seat of My Pants

Shortly after I went to work for the Band in 1989, it opened a sub-office in Prince George to improve communications between the Band and outside agencies. Phone communications from Fort Ware were so poor as to be almost non-existent, although they improved somewhat when Jim Van Somer installed his radio phone, which was relayed through Vancouver, in the late 1960s. In 1986, Northwest Tel took over the communications system and constructed a large satellite dish and computerized telephone switchboard that connected with Fort Nelson. People in Fort Ware started to get phones installed in their homes and with the ease that calls could be made, the system was well used—that is, until the first telephone bills arrived in the mail with expensive long distance calls on their accounts. Many subscribers soon had the phones removed.

The cost of flying people in and out of Fort Ware for meetings with government agencies was prohibitive. The office in Prince George solved both problems and provided a communications base for the Band and an office for me to work in. At the beginning I worked in that office about three weeks a month and spent the other week in Fort Ware. The amount of time I spent in Fort Ware gradually increased though and some years later I was spending the three weeks there and just one week in Prince George.

Besides initiating changes in radio communication, Jim Van Somer also directed the construction of a rough airstrip in the late 1970s to the north of the village on a relatively level piece of high ground. There were no buildings close by that would be a hazard for the planes landing because the old Hudson's Bay store that had once stood on the riverbank had been dismantled years previously. All that remained was a stone chimney at the bottom of the bank where the manager's residence and storehouse had been. A new growth of spruce and willow now covered the area that had seen so much activity at the turn of the twentieth century. A small new store had been constructed near to a water tower but both were located over to the side of the flight path that planes would be using.

I was asked to fly up to Fort Ware from Prince George on a regularly scheduled plane operated by Northern Thunderbird Air, which flew either a Beechcraft 18 twin-engine plane or a Beaver on wheels or skis. The Beaver is often referred to as the workhorse of the north and is the most common bush plane in northern Canada. Both planes were slow and noisy but quite often I was able to ride in the co-pilot's seat where I had a great view of the countryside far below us, and I could talk to the pilot using a spare headset and microphone.

Whenever I visited Fort Ware, I met with the Chief and his Council and discussed various government programs with them, finding what they wanted to do and assessing what we would be able to do with our limited resources. Then I spent my time back in Prince George trying to put their ideas on paper and attending meetings with various government departments to try and put the programs into effect, usually requesting funding for them. Chief McCook was quite blunt about his attitude to government and he was very forthright about playing the "dumb Indian" when he wanted something from the government. Government bureaucrats would feel sorry for him and then usually agree to his requests, bending over backwards to help him.

The people in Fort Ware were used to gathering specific foods at specific times in the year and their lives still revolved around some of these traditional activities so the precise time of day was not very important to them. On one occasion, just before I became Band Manager, I came to realize that for Chief Emil McCook and his Council, time was relative. I had flown into Fort Ware on a prearranged date to meet with the Chief. When I arrived by charter airplane, I went to his office but he wasn't there. I asked where I could find him. "Oh, he went hunting this morning and didn't know when he'd be back," was the reply. I was a little annoyed by this and thought that my trip was a waste of my time and government money.

"Didn't he remember about our meeting?" I asked, trying to suppress my annoyance.

"Well, I know that he was out of meat and some boys saw moose tracks up the White [the Kwadacha River], so he went after them," was the explanation.

I went off in a bit of a huff to eat my lunch and as I bit into my sandwich I suddenly thought about what I would do if I had nothing to eat. I realized that, as far as Emil was concerned, our meeting could take place at any time and the money that I had spent chartering a plane was not my own money, it was "government money." Food for him and his family, on the other hand, was of paramount importance, so he did the obvious thing when he heard that moose had been seen a few miles away—he went off to hunt them. (Moose was part of the staple diet of most of the First Nations people in Fort Ware.)

This attitude to time was also displayed when I went to meetings in the city with Emil. He would dawdle and look in store windows at things that interested him and I was always worried that he might take it into his mind to call in at a pub on the way to a meeting to bolster his confidence. If he had too many drinks, he would be "dizzy," a term commonly used in Fort Ware for someone who had "been into his cups" or was inebriated by homebrew. I would be anxiously scanning my watch every few seconds, but most times we arrived in whatever office we were headed for on time or very close to it, and I was always surprised at how willingly people accommodated this well-known Band Chief from an isolated northern tribe.

I continued to travel to Fort Ware on a regular basis, but one day I paid a very unexpected visit to the village. I was not due to visit Fort Ware for another couple of weeks and I was in the office in Prince George doing some much-needed paperwork and waiting for lunchtime, when I had arranged to meet my wife at a local restaurant.

Earlier that morning, we had chartered the Beech 18 from Northern Thunderbird Air to send eight Fort Ware Band members back to their village after they had been to various medical appointments. About 10:30 in the morning, I received a call from the airline to say that they had a problem with the passengers, most of whom had been drinking all night or early that morning. The pilot, Lester Bower, was taxiing down the runway ready for take-off when one large, belligerent woman decided that she wanted to get off the plane. She undid her seat belt and climbed out of her seat. Lester immediately abandoned his flight plan and returned to the airline base.

My office phone rang.

"Unless someone from the office comes to control these guys, the flight is off!"

"Do you mean get a policeman?"

"No, just have someone come along and keep them in their seats."

I did not have to guess which "someone" Lester had in mind because I don't think that keeping the peace in a plane full of drunks was in the secretary's job description. I said I would come up to the airport and discuss it.

Northern Thunderbird Air was quite within its rights to refuse to fly, but if we did not get the people back home, I knew that no hotel in town would take them in an inebriated state. I thought that maybe reading the riot act to them might make a difference. Ha! I arrived at the airport and spoke to the people. Of course, they immediately agreed to behave and then started arguing amongst themselves about who had caused the trouble before. They started getting rowdy again, so I could see I would have to go along for the ride. I phoned my wife to say, "Sorry, love, I can't have lunch with you because I am flying to Fort Ware to look after some rowdy Band members!"—or words to that effect.

I sat in the back of the Beechcraft where I could see everyone, and we soon continued north with a lot of noise, both from the aircraft and the passengers. We had almost reached McLeod Lake when the man sitting to my right held out a large bottle and said, "Keith, do you want some of this wine?"

I groaned and told him to put it away. He didn't. Instead, he began to pass the bottle around and it travelled from person to person. The whole plane reeked of sweet wine, but at least everyone stayed in their seats. We were halfway up Williston Lake when the woman who had been belligerent earlier shouted at me to tell the pilot to land because she wanted to go to the bathroom really bad. I told her that we were flying over the middle of the lake and there was nowhere to land, she would have to wait, but no, she was insistent that the plane land and proceeded to get up from her seat.

"I'll tell him that he'd better land or else!" she exclaimed.

I grabbed the back of her pants and hauled her back into her seat. "There is nowhere to land around here. We have gone past all the logging camps," I told her. I was lying, because I knew there was actually a landing strip on the east side of the lake, but there was no way I was going to ask Lester to try to land there.

The woman struggled up again and again I hauled her back.

"Give me that wine bottle," I asked my neighbour and he willingly passed it over.

"Here, I'll give you a drink, if you'll just sit down." I passed her a small paper cupful and she relaxed in her seat. It was three-quarters of an hour later and a few more cups of wine—some of which were tipped over me—before we reached Fort Ware and landed. The inebriated passengers were unloaded, and I moved to the co-pilot's seat for the return journey, smelling like a winery.

Lester, the pilot, and I travelled back to Prince George in relative peace and comfort and then I phoned my wife again to tell her about my recent escapade. Lester was very understanding and sympathetic, but safety was his main concern and no one from Fort Ware ever held a grudge against him if he refused to let them fly.

I could see that working for this Band was going to be quite challenging.

Listen to the Band

Chief Emil McCook asked me to accompany him to various meetings throughout the province in my role as Band Manager. Sometimes we went to the Yukon when he and the Council met with the Kaska Dene Tribal Council. Fort Ware was a member band of this tribal council.

The Rocky Mountain Trench runs diagonally from the southeast to the northwest of British Columbia, with towering mountains on either side. It is a place where long ago two geological plates came together, forcing the land to heave and leaving a fault line to scar the landscape. Although the mountains we call the Rocky Mountains end in northern BC, the fault line continues through the Liard Plain and into the Yukon, running northwest with the Welwyn Mountains to the northeast and the Dawson Range to the southwest. The fault line running from Watson Lake to Dawson City is called the Tintina Trench.

The whole central area is now the homeland of the Kaska Dene, from Ross River to Upper Liard in the Yukon to Lower Post, Good Hope Lake and Fort Ware in British Columbia. The Kaska and Sekani people regularly travelled up and down the trench on centuries-old trails, searching out the means for survival.

Many years ago, the Fort Ware Band joined the Carrier Sekani Tribal Council in Prince George to negotiate their land claim, but after several years, the Band Council decided this was not the best organization for them and withdrew. Later, they joined the Kaska Dene Tribal Council to negotiate their land claim. The Chief of the Fort Ware Band at the time, Emil McCook, was a Kaska man, and he felt that the Fort Ware people were of Kaska origin. According to some band members, however, they consist of a mixture of Sekani and Kaska people.

Land claims talks with the federal and provincial governments are ongoing at the time of writing and the Kaska have been continually asked to prove their claim to the land that they say they have been using for hundreds of years. The Fort Ware Band takes part in these hearings as part of the Kaska Tribal Council, along with southern Yukon bands. Because the Kaska people have land on either side of the BC-Yukon border, negotiations are difficult. They require a meeting of the minds of the different governments—the federal, BC and Yukon governments, plus the Kaska Tribal Council government. Land use is a major factor in the land claims negotiations, and the umbilical cord that connects the Fort Ware Band, now known as the Kwadacha Nation, to the rest of the Kaska is the Davie Trail, which runs 460 kilometres up the Rocky Mountain Trench from Fort Ware to Lower Post, another First Nations village just inside the BC border and just south of Watson Lake in the Yukon.

The Fort Ware Band is also greatly concerned with the logging that is taking place along the Rocky Mountain Trench. It has been undertaken in a big way and the people are alarmed to see their hills and mountains denuded of trees. After Williston Lake was created, logging debris clogged the mouth of the Finlay River and made it impassable by boat. As a result of the logging activity, the prices for food and fuel became extremely high because they had to be flown into the village by charter aircraft. The Fort Ware people felt angry, frustrated and helpless.

The Band has gradually become more aware of the value of the land, especially the timber and subsurface minerals, with the potential for oil and gas revenue, all of it claimed by the provincial government. The Band Council found this untenable and felt they could not stand by and see millions of dollars going south while they themselves lived in poverty. It was into such situations that I was gradually immersed by the Chief and Council while the Kaska Dene Tribal Council worked with the Band to try to find ways to mitigate these economic problems and settle the land claims.

Every year the Kaska Tribal Council holds a general assembly where reports of the various member bands' activities during the past year are presented and proposals for the future are discussed and decided upon. The assemblies are held in different places in Kaska territory and I was able to attend them all, whether they were held at Frances Lake in the Yukon or Rapid River in northern British Columbia. One that was especially enjoyable and relaxing was held at Liard Hot Springs on the Alaska Highway.

Each year a different member band sponsored the assembly. When Fort Ware hosted it, a site about twenty kilometres south of Fort Ware was chosen. There the forestry department, along with a mining company, had built a long, wide gravel airstrip at what was then called Finbow. There was a bend in the Finlay River like a reverse "D" and the airstrip was built on the flat land in the crook of the river. (Later the name was changed to "Buffalo Head," for some strange reason.)

I bought all the groceries and supplies for the assembly and drove everything up in a rented trailer. We arranged to rent a cook shack from one of the logging camps and brought it to the site. Louise Van Somer, Jim's wife, was hired as the chief cook and half a dozen local people were hired to help her. Shelters were erected for the meetings, and campsites cleared. By the time the assembly started, I was worn out.

These assemblies were quite inspiring and I was able to see Native government at its best. Most of the day was spent in meetings held in a large, specially constructed tent frame made of poles covered with tarps or plastic. Just outside this shelter, a huge fire was kept burning and on it a grill sat with a cauldron of coffee and a huge kettle of tea.

The Tribal Chief, Hammond Dick, started the day with a drum beat broadcast over a loudspeaker system. When all the Chiefs were present, the meeting was opened with a prayer from one of the Elders, said in their own language.

When the business end of the day was over, people relaxed and visited old friends and distant relatives until supper was served. Dinner was quite a task for the women of the host Band, who had to cook and serve nearly three hundred people.

It wasn't long after dinner before the drums would start and stick gambling would begin. Wood smoke hung over the campsite and permeated everything, a not-too-unpleasant smell out in the wilderness—plus it helped keep the flies and mosquitoes at bay. In the flickering light of the campfires, people watched the teams, laughing and cheering on their favourites. Others sat around their campfires and either listened or shared gossip with friends.

Gambling seems like a national pastime for the many First Nations people that I have observed and stick gambling is one of the Sekani and Kaska social highlights. It usually takes place with a certain amount of seriousness but also much good humour and, to the casual observer, it looks like a group game of sleight of hand. Stick gambling usually begins in the late afternoon and goes on well into the night, accompanied by the rhythmic drumming and singing of five or six young men, which seems to work the players and the audience up to fever pitch. At the end of a game, there is much shouting and laughing and everyone relaxes again.

Early one summer in 1988, I had the privilege of being invited, along with the people of Fort Ware, to the General Assembly of the Kaska Dena, which was hosted by the Kaska people of Ross River in the Yukon. In a letter that I sent home to my wife, I wrote the following:

> It's nine thirty in the evening and I am at a small lake close to Ross River in the Yukon Territory. The sun will be setting in about an hour and the few wisps of cloud will almost disappear into the dusk, almost, because it doesn't really get dark this far north at this time of the year.
>
> I can smell wood smoke from the many campfires around the lake and it smells sweet on the evening breeze. The blue smoke drifts slowly through the clumps of spruce on the north end of the lake and disappears against the grey mountains on the southwest horizon, and as if a perfect climax was needed, a loon's call echoed around the lake. This is no regular campsite, and I can't make up my mind if I am very fortunate to be here, or am I living a make believe life?
>
> At the moment there is a lull in the drumming and singing while the drummers hold their caribou hide drums close to the fire to tighten them. A few moments ago their rhythmic drumming and singing could be heard coming from the main gathering place where a large fire burned, and on the ground in front of the drummers, two lines of men knelt down facing each other, and as they swayed to the rhythm of the drums, one team first held their hands behind their backs and then, with a grand flourish they brought their hands in front of them, some

crossing their arms, and all of the time rocking backwards and forwards, up and down, to the incessant and persistent beat of the ten drums.

Suddenly, a man on the opposing team leans forward, claps his hands together, then with his left hand pointing at one of the opposing team members, he then indicates with his right thumb, so that all the opposing team members to the right of the one he had pointed at, all have to open one of their hands to either reveal a quarter, perhaps a stone, or maybe, to whoops of laughter and general mayhem, an empty palm! The ones who are caught with an object in their hand throw a stick to the other team, and this goes on until the one team has all the sticks. I guess that's why it is called "stick gambling"! One of these days I will figure out the intricacies of the game and report back!

The People at the End of the Rocks

First Nations people living in the northern interior of British Columbia were hardy people. They had to be to survive in the harsh environment. In their need to find food, they had to be semi-nomadic and consequently walked long distances to the areas where seasonal foods could be found. Mountains were no obstacle. Indeed, they were the source of most of the food, and climbing mountains was not considered something to be avoided.

The people who lived in the area of Fort Grahame, which now lies deep below the surface of Williston Lake, were called "Tsay-keh-ne-az" in the Sekani dialect. This means "The Little People of the Rocks." The Sekani people who lived farther north in the Fort Ware area were referred to as the "Tse-loh-ne"—"The People at the End of the Rocks." The rocks referred to are probably the Rocky Mountains, which end at Terminus Mountain, over two hundred kilometres north of Fort Ware and halfway up the Davie Trail. These "people of the rocks" travelled frequently along a vast network of established trails that ran throughout their territory, walking hundreds of kilometres annually.

Until quite recently, whole families would travel to the Omenica and Rocky Mountains in the summertime, hoping to hunt some mountain sheep or a few ptarmigan. The animal they most sought in the old days, however, was the marmot, a fairly large, rock-dwelling rodent, whose tender fatty flesh was desired by all—including the numerous grizzly bears that also frequented the mountains and who would tear great boulders apart in their quest for this quarry. The bears had their own coats to keep them warm, but the Native people wanted both the meat and the fur for coats and blankets.

Simon Fraser, a fur trader for the North West Company, and Samuel Black, who worked for the Hudson's Bay Company, both travelled in Sekani country, "discovering" it as far as Britain was concerned. They described how the Sekani followed well-established trails, harvesting their food as they went. Sometimes they camped for a long time at a fishing lake in the summertime. These travellers reported that the Sekani left the mountains in late summer to hunt buffalo and moose on the eastern side of the Rockies, but they were not always successful, because the Beaver and Cree controlled the hunting in that area and the Sekani were pushed west. In some accounts, the Sekani were said to live in fear of the more aggressive Cree to the east, the Carrier to the south and other tribes to the west. When Alexander Mackenzie, another North West Company trader, met a family of Sekani in 1793, they were trading beaver pelts with the Carrier Nation. It seems that, because they were surrounded by potential enemies, the Sekani moved or were pushed into the Rocky Mountain Trench, which was considered too unproductive for other Aboriginal peoples to desire.

In 1797, John Finlay, after whom the Finlay River was named, travelled up the Finlay with much difficulty as far as Ingenika Forks, before turning back because of the turbulent, log-laden waters. He was guided by a party of "Sikannis," a group that included two "Sikanni" women who carried most of the freight on game trails along the side of the Finlay River while the men lined their birchbark canoe up the fast-flowing river through narrow canyons and waterfalls. Lining a canoe meant tying a rope to the canoe while one man pulled it up against the current and another man with a paddle kept the canoe from coming too close to the bank, where it could be damaged by the rocks. Sometimes, when the way was too difficult, they would carry the canoe over the rocks and then go back for their belongings.

There was a difference of opinion among these white explorers about the abundance of food or lack of it in the Rocky Mountain Trench. Perhaps this was because the animals move around seasonally, or it may have been the weather in a particular year, or even just the vagaries of animal populations. Samuel Black, for instance, found the upper Finlay to be "a barren waste, scanty of subsistence." He was, of course, looking for country that would bring in lots of fur so that a Hudson's Bay outpost could be established there. In contrast, the anthropologist Diamond Jenness reported that the Sekani relied on the abundant wild animals and spoke of the headwaters of the Finlay as being amongst the finest game areas in all of North America. Today the world-famous lodges in the Rocky Mountain Trench at Scoop Lake and Terminus Mountain boast about the number of wild animals in the area and the creation of the Muskwa-Kechika Special Management area attests to the latter view as well. Yet my personal observation has been that at different times of the year there is a dearth of animals in some areas and an abundance of them at other times.

Non-aboriginal travellers were very aware of the nomadic nature of the Sekani and for decades it was a source of frustration to the Hudson's Bay Company, which wished to attach Indians to particular posts so that they would be sure that furs would be brought in to pay off the debts incurred when a Native family was "grubstaked" for the trapping season. An old patriarch of the Fort Ware Band, Aatse Davie—for whom the Davie Trail is named—did not want any part of this association with one particular post. He knew that if his people did not live on the land there would be disastrous consequences for his family. Diamond Jenness reported that Davie only stayed by a trading post long enough to sell his furs, never intermingling with the people who lived around the store. He felt that if his family mixed with others, they would "crave for an idler life which would sap the energies of his people and induce them to remain [around the store]." For a time, the Band members were left to their hunting and fishing, and seemed to have been forgotten by the rest of the country. Consequently, seasonal travel by First Nations people continued without hindrance up and down the Rocky Mountain Trench on the Davie Trail.

Davie didn't only walk up and down the Trench on his search for food and furs, as countless generations of his ancestors had done long before there was a Lower Post or Fort Grahame. He also walked west, through Spatsizi country to the Iskut River, then north, following the Dease River, then farther north to Frances Lake in the Yukon. He also walked—or rather climbed—through the Kwadacha Mountains to the northeast of Fort Ware.

It was said that Davie (whose Christian name was Hamilton—a name that never seemed to get used), ruled his Band with complete authority, like a "Hebrew patriarch," according to an anthropological bulletin written by Diamond Jenness. Jenness also said that this Band, at that time called the T'lotona or Long Grass Indians, "was remarkably free from disease that had attacked surrounding Indians; the adults were well clad, the children clean and healthy." Davie and his family (he had four daughters) kept very much to themselves. He chose husbands for his daughters very carefully, many of them of Kaska origin, and so his family grew. By 1924, when Davie was an old man in his seventies, there were forty members in his family band.

Old Davie—the "old" was a mark of respect and honour—was called Aatse Davie in the Sekani language. This really meant "Grandfather Davie."

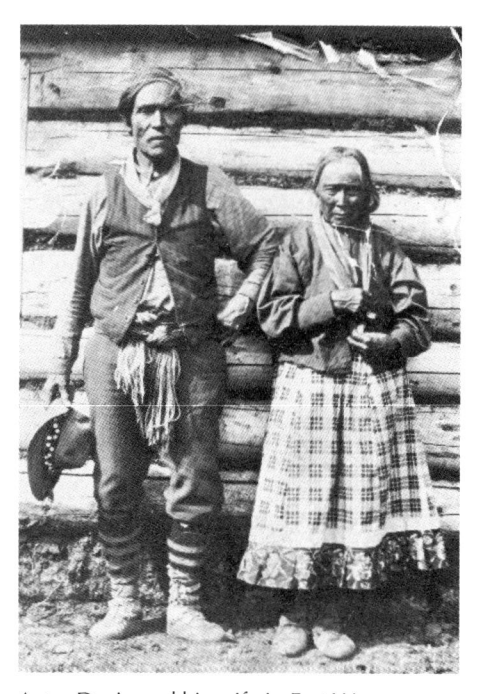

Aatse Davie and his wife in Fort Ware.

He was a strong leader of men, the son of a French-Canadian trapper and a Native woman of mixed ancestry from the Tseloni and the Sasuchan people of the Bear Lake area northeast of Takla Landing. According to Adrien Gabriel Morice, a Jesuit priest and noted First Nations historian, and anthropologist Diamond Jenness, the Sasuchan that Davie's mother belonged to had intermarried with the Gitxsan and then moved to Fort Grahame on the Finlay River. However, it was because of his wife's heritage as a Finlay River woman, that Davie had hunting rights up the Rocky Mountain Trench.

Dressed like most people of his era, he usually wore a western hat over his medium-length hair. When he removed his hat, it could be seen that he combed it over his scalp from left to right. He wore a cloth vest or "waistcoat" over his shirt, and around his neck was a kerchief. A fringed sash was worn around his waist and hung down the front of his wool pants, which were tucked inside his calf-high moccasins. He was tall and slim and had a confident look on his sombre face. Like other people who travel and work hard in the bush, Aatse Davie's size and looks belied the stamina of this remarkable man.

The Sekani people of the region traditionally gathered annually at the confluence of the Fox, Kwadacha and Finlay rivers where Fort Ware is now situated. They would trade, tell stories and, no doubt, play many gambling games. The young people would look for and find mates and old friendships would be renewed. Communication among the families was possible because the Kaska and Sekani languages are very closely related. They are both Athapascan in origin, and different dialects of the Tsek'eni (Sekani) language is spoken at many of the northern villages, including Tseh Keh, McLeod Lake, Takla Landing and Iskut, demonstrating the historic relationships that exist among the bands. Others have said that the Beaver and Cree languages were also understandable and Chief Emil McCook told me he could understand people from other villages as long as they spoke slowly—but if they got excited and spoke quickly, he lost the gist of the conversation.

When the Hudson's Bay Company, always on the lookout for furs, finally opened an outpost in 1927, it chose this traditional gathering place, where the Kwadacha River enters the Finlay River. They named it Whitewater Post, but when a post office was established in the village in 1938, the name was changed to Fort Ware. This name was registered by the Department of Indian Affairs. It was named for William Ware, the manager of the Hudson's Bay Company BC district from 1927 to 1932.

When R.G. McConnell of the Canadian Geologic Survey travelled up much of the Finlay River in 1893, he reported that "native Sekanni travelled through the upper Finlay region but did not have any permanent residences there." But, as seemed to happen all over the north—and just as Old Davie had feared—people began to stay around the Hudson's Bay post, where rations of tea and sugar were more readily available and where, even more important in the eyes of the adults, they could trade furs for plugs of chewing tobacco. Old Davie's descendants did not have the discipline that the patriarch had and slowly they gravitated to the store, where they spent increasingly more of their time.

Although most of the land is officially considered Crown land today, to the First Nations people it is, and has always been, their land. In the past, it supplied them with everything they needed to survive—food, clothing and shelter—as they roamed over their vast territory. The original inhabitants travelled over this land for thousands of years before the white explorers came, and evidence of the trails they travelled on for countless years still criss-crosses the northern interior of British Columbia.

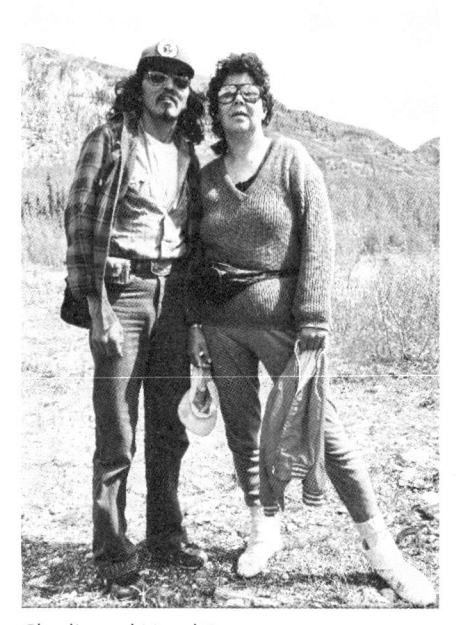

Charlie and Hazel Boya.

Simon Fraser, Alexander Mackenzie, and more recently, Frank Swannell and others, have received credit for discovering and mapping waterways and exploring the interior of British Columbia, but they did not do it alone. Very little acknowledgment was given to the people who guided them along well-worn trails and warned them of rapids and whirlpools that were dangerous for small boat travel. Then they stood by silently as these intruders gave strange names to what were to them familiar rivers and mountains.

Lheitli Tenneh Chief Peter Quaw, at a meeting some years ago with Justice Thomas Berger, famous for conducting the Berger Pipeline Inquiry, stated that: "We are programmed to believe that Columbus discovered America, even though millions of people were living there already!"

In keeping with modern thinking, and wishing to assert their individuality, the Fort Ware Band changed its name to one that they felt identified them in their own language. In 1998, after much deliberation, the Chief and his Council decided to call the band the Kwadacha Band after the name of the river that runs from the rugged mountains northeast from its source in Kwadacha Wilderness Provincial Park and empties its pale, silty waters into the Finlay River at Fort Ware. Fort Ware itself is now sometimes called Kwadacha.

Kwadacha is a Sekani word that is difficult to translate into English. One Elder told me that it means "somebody hiding something there" or "something big." Patterson, in his book *Finlay's River*, translates it as "big white water," and Fort Ware Elder Minnie McCook called the river "The White," because in the springtime the water looks white with all of the glacial silt that is carried from the mountains to the east. When Charles Bedaux travelled down the White/Kwadacha River in the 1930s, his map shows Fort Ware as "Whitewater." It seems a strange twist that most of the

Fort Ware people still refer to the river as the "White," a non-Native name, even though topographical maps have always labelled it the "Kwadacha," the First Nations name.

Maps of British Columbia show a dotted line running from Watson Lake in the Yukon, down to Fort Ware, still the most isolated village in British Columbia. The dotted line represents the 460-kilometre Davie Trail, called Aatse Dene Tunna by the Kaska Nation in their language. Although this trail is hardly known outside of Fort Ware today, its history as a traditional trail is fascinating. It is long and arduous, situated in the middle of some spectacular country. Very few people get to see this area and it was an honour for me to be invited to accompany Charlie and Hazel Boya on this intriguing historical trail. I hoped to satisfy my curiosity about the country, the people and the history surrounding its use by the Sekani and other pioneers.

Take a Walk

As time passed, fewer non-Native people travelled through Aatse Davie's old haunts and the land remained virtually untouched. The Davie Trail is not used in its entirety today and you could count on one hand the few intrepid summer hikers who dare to tempt mosquitoes and blackflies to attack their sweaty bodies as they travel down the trail. The route, its isolation and its history make it a worthwhile challenge for those very few hardy adventurers.

The trail does not see many First Nations people on it these days, either, except for a few Fort Ware residents like Charlie and Hazel Boya and their family, who spend time at their cabin at Terminus Mountain, two hundred kilometres north of Fort Ware. There are a few local hunters who might travel north for thirty or forty kilometres from Fort Ware and some Kaska hunters who travel south from Lower Post for sixty or seventy kilometres.

Sometime in the 1970s, a group of Fort Ware men travelled east over the Rocky Mountains to the Halfway River Reserve following another of the old trails. They brought a small herd of horses back with them. I was told that it was a tough trip for both men and horses but instead of coming down the Kwadacha River, which empties into the Finlay River at Fort Ware, they came down to the Finlay River by way of the Akie River just south of Fort Ware, a route that was easier on the horses. I was also told that besides getting horses one young man, who had always seemed shy, found himself a beautiful young woman in Halfway whom he married and brought back to Fort Ware.

There has been some effort by a few people in Fort Ware to open the trail with a view to attracting hardy adventure tourists, and as part of the local Justice Committee recommendations, young male offenders have been sentenced to work on such projects as trail-clearing and cabin-building. These activities are far more productive than incarcerating them in a correctional facility down south. Some of these young men have not had the opportunity to travel very far in their homeland because their parents had ceased to live out in the bush.

There are also seasonal hunters who fly in and use segments of the Davie Trail under the watchful eye of hunting guides, but this only happens for a few weeks at a time during the hunting season. Most of these hunters stay at Scoop Lake, Terminus Mountain and other lodges where outfitters have "fly camps"—small cabins scattered around in the mountains and valleys where the hunting is good.

The Davie Trail has thus been left in part to a few Native trappers at either end of the trail and the guide outfitters, but mostly it has been left to the large game animals that abound in this wilderness area and seldom see any sign of man anymore. Consequently, the Davie Trail has almost reverted to its natural state.

As First Nations people try to document their heritage for land claims negotiations, northern trails research has contributed to a cultural awakening, especially for the young people, as they became more aware of their history. A project to document the history of the people while there are still a few Elders alive who remember the land as it was many years ago is underway under the direction of the Aatse Davie School in Fort Ware. Ms. Susan Hatfield-McCook from the College of New Caledonia in Prince George gathers the Elders together at the Aatse Davie School whenever possible so they can sit and recall times past.

One Elder from Fort Ware, Minnie McCook, the adopted granddaughter of Aatse Davie, walked many hundreds of miles every year—wherever Davie took the family. After she married John McCook, who became Chief of the Band, she continued to travel up and down the Davie Trail, a part of which served as John McCook's trapline. One time when I was out on my snowmobile visiting cabins north of Fort Ware, I met Minnie out on the trail miles from anywhere and asked her where she was going.

"Oh, I'm just looking for some chicken," she said with a smile. (Chicken is what most First Nations people called a grouse.) She then indicated her .22 rifle. "This gun, it's old like me, but it shoots good."

With these words, she set off down the trail. A few hours later, I went to her daughter Hazel's house and there was Minnie sitting drinking tea, not looking the least bit tired! I was so surprised to see her there that I forgot to ask her if she had shot any "chickens."

Minnie rarely sat around, even when she was almost ninety years old. Always there to help anyone in need, she conveyed the air of a gentle aristocrat. Her daughter Hazel laughingly told me that back in Fort Ware, Minnie often said she was going out to visit "those old people" in the village, even though many, if not most of them, were younger than she was!

Hazel Boya was the daughter of John and Minnie McCook and though Hazel had lived in Fort Ware some of the time, she had spent most of her formative years in various trapping cabins along the Davie Trail where she was taught by her bush-wise father to hunt and shoot a rifle. She also learned about natural healing and herb remedies from her mother, and how to skin beaver and make moose dry-meat, a couple of the daily chores performed by her quiet, unassuming mother.

Another diminutive old lady, Angela McCook, now in her eighties and, at the time of writing, still living in Fort Ware, remembers that as a teenager she walked many times from Fort Grahame along a part of the Davie Trail. She would branch over to the west following the Finlay River, walk past the Fishing Lakes and through what is now Spatsizi Park over to Iskut village, and then north to

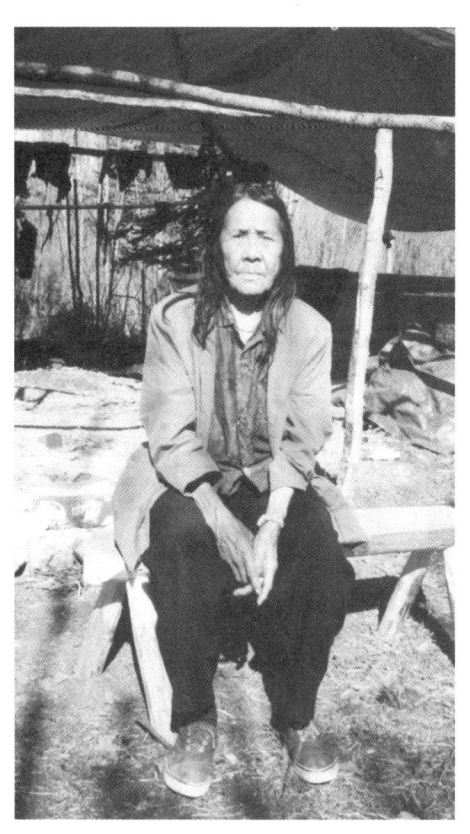

Hazel Boya's mother, Minnie McCook.

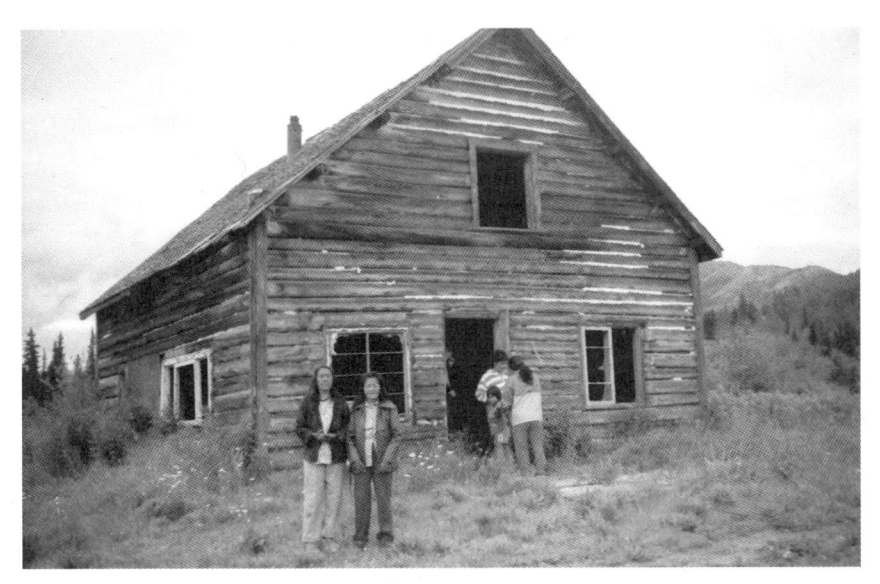

Minnie McCook at the old Bay store in McDames.

McDames on the Dease River. There she and her family stayed for a while before going on to Lower Post, then back down the Davie Trail to the Finlay River once again—a distance of well over eight hundred kilometres. Another route went north and west through Fox Pass, and then followed a valley that ran parallel to the Omenica Mountains to spectacular Oboe Lake. Walking these trails was a normal and accepted part of life that continued on into the 1960s.

Charlie Boya

There are people who can sit around all day and watch other people work, and then there are people like Hazel's husband, Charlie Boya. In his knowledge of the northern environment, animal behaviour, his survival abilities and stamina, Charlie is like a reincarnated Aatse Davie. From morning until evening, Charlie is like a wound-up spring, his long black hair, tied in a ponytail, whisking behind him as his lean, muscular frame takes him from project to project at a hurried pace that would tire most people out by the end of the day.

Unlike some Fort Ware residents, who never made any improvements to their houses or yards, Charlie Boya built a log fence around his house and planted grass seed, but all the while, he said, both he and his wife Hazel dreamed of their little trapping cabin at Terminus Mountain.

When I first met Charlie Boya in the 1970s, he was preparing to travel up the Davie Trail by dog team in early winter with Hazel and their daughter, Caroline. They were heading for his trapline. They had a log cabin halfway up the Rocky Mountain Trench on the eastern bank of the Kechika River at Terminus Mountain and they were going to spend the rest of the winter there.

It was a journey of 230 kilometres as the crow flies from Fort Ware to their cabin. It is 630 kilometres north of Prince George in central British Columbia and more than 1,600 kilometres from Vancouver. When I asked

Charlie how long it would take him to reach Terminus Mountain, he just shrugged and replied with a smile that it would take as long as it took to get there. Time was not important and there were a few cabins on the way where the family could stay, he said, or he would just fasten some tarpaulins up between some trees, build a large fire, and camp. He had done it before, and he was quite confident that he, his wife and their young daughter would be quite comfortable and safe.

Charlie was then in his late twenties, married, with just the one daughter. When I spoke to him, he was busy on the bank of the Finlay River harnessing four pathetic-looking sled dogs to a heavily loaded toboggan. This was not a toboggan like those that children buy from a department store, but a hand-made wooden toboggan about three metres long and forty-five centimetres wide. Handlebars were attached at the back for the driver to help guide, and at times, push the toboggan when the dogs were tired or when they encountered a steep hill. The toboggan sat on two runners, or skis, and when the trail was well used and hard packed, the toboggan could glide easily along. The driver stood on the runners and would then kick one leg just like a child does to move a scooter along the road. Passengers were sometimes carried in the toboggan or they sat on top of the load, ready to jump off if necessary, to walk behind and give the dogs some relief.

I had driven dog teams hundreds of kilometres in the western Arctic for over six years and in British Columbia for over fifteen years and was used to seeing large husky dogs pulling heavy oak toboggans loaded with firewood or caribou meat or a whole winter camping outfit. I thought to myself that here I was in Fort Ware in northern British Columbia looking at an apology for a dog team. In my opinion, this young man was not going to get far with this outfit.

This goes to show how little I knew about Charlie Boya, his wife, Hazel, or the Davie Trail.

I knew that most of my perceptions of life in the bush were rather romantic compared to what was, in reality, a very hard life. After Charlie and Hazel Boya married, they lived mainly in Fort Ware. They felt that if their children—they eventually had six, two boys and four girls, and also looked after two grandchildren—were to have any future, Charlie would have to take a role in the leadership of the Sekani community in Fort Ware. So he ran for Chief of the Band in the biennial elections with the vigorous support of Hazel, who, after all, was the daughter of a highly esteemed Chief, John McCook, which gave Hazel some prestige in the

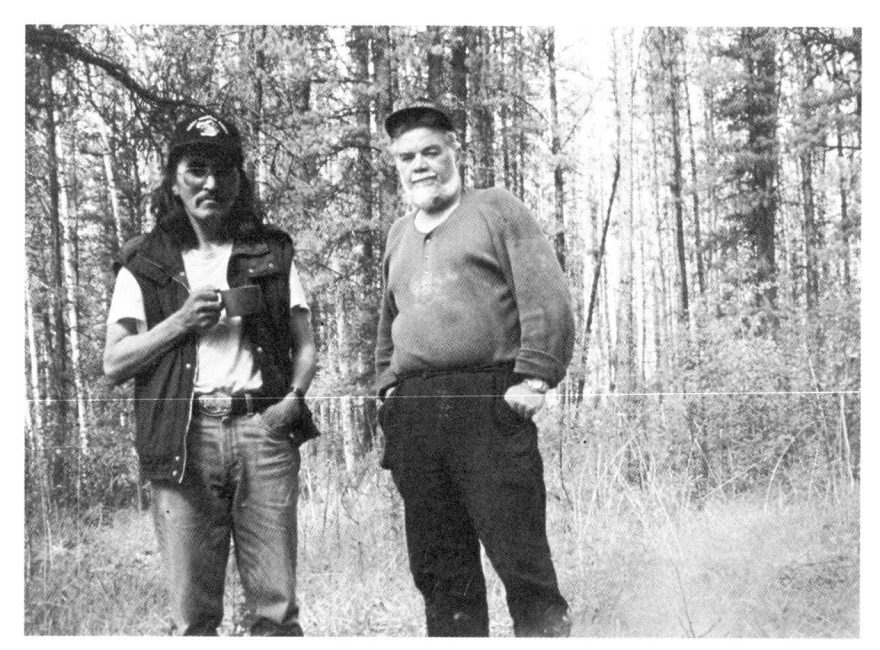

Charlie Boya, left, and Keith take a trail break.

community. Having Aatse Davie as her great-grandfather certainly would have helped too.

Hazel was a respected Sekani woman, who was quietly spoken like her mother, Minnie McCook, but if she felt strongly about something or, worse, if she was opposed to something that was happening in the village, you could see the fire in her eyes and hear it in her voice. Charlie and Hazel made a formidable team and to everyone's surprise, in the election, Charlie unseated Emil McCook, who had been Chief for over twenty-seven years. The *BC Report* magazine quoted the new Chief Charlie Boya as saying that he promised to "hold fast to the principle that leadership and booze don't mix." In spite of Charlie's zeal, he was dogged by tragedy and experienced two major family crises during the period that he was Chief.

In the first instance, Charlie and Hazel's son, Jonathan, was involved in two separate accidents. In the first one, his eyesight was severely damaged. He suffered another, more serious injury when he was thrown off his snowmobile and fractured his spine, which rendered him a quadriplegic. After a prolonged period in the G.F. Strong rehabilitation hospital in Vancouver, he was able to return to live in Prince George with partial use of his hands. Charlie and Hazel had barely recovered from this blow when their daughter,

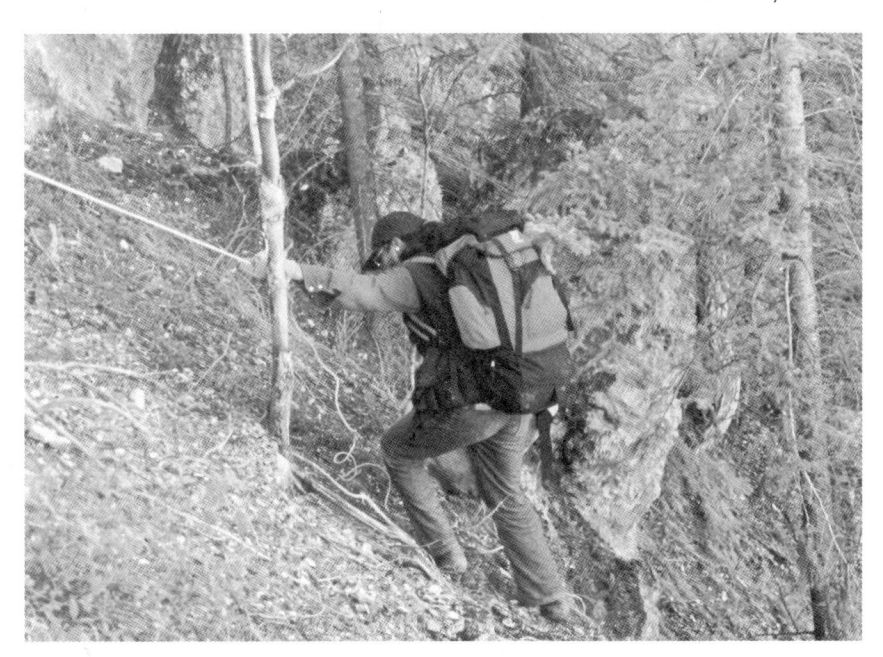

A real cliffhanger: Charlie Boya navigates a rough part of the trail.

Lila, died suddenly from a prescription medicine overdose, and the grieving parents could not be comforted.

In despair, Charlie refused to run for a second term in office and vowed that he would take his remaining family out of the village and live at Terminus Mountain again. But the need to keep in close contact with his injured son made this too difficult and, realizing that his other children needed the benefit of an education, he reluctantly lived in the village, although he continued to travel periodically with his family to a cabin that he had built some years previously at Fox Lake, sixty-five kilometres north of Fort Ware.

This cabin had been built so that Charlie and Hazel could visit Hazel's father, John McCook, when he was still alive, and who also had a log cabin on a quiet bay on Fox Lake. He and Minnie had lived there for part of every year when he was trapping. John McCook died in 1988 and Minnie then moved to Fort Ware, where she died in 2010.

At the next village election, Emil McCook was re-elected as the Chief and he and Charlie always remained on good terms.

As the years passed, Charlie and I became firm friends and I was always welcome in his house. When I went to the village when I was first employed by the Band, and needed somewhere to stay, I stayed in the cabin Charlie had built in his fenced-off area, and I had many opportunities to visit in the evenings. He loved to tease and joke and most of the time I seemed to be on the receiving end of his jokes.

Charlie referred to me less and less as a white man and used to joke to others about how I was almost Kaska (the linguistic group to which he had belonged when he was a boy in Lower Post). I took this as a compliment and after travelling through the northern country with Charlie and Hazel, he remarked that I had seen more of Kaska country than many of the young First Nations people. Usually in the wintertime, I travelled to Charlie's Fox Lake cabin, travelling by snowmobile over frozen lakes and through the deep snow in the bush. Once or twice I travelled the sixty-four kilometres on my own, using snowshoes to break trail when my snowmobile got stuck in the deep drifts. I always enjoyed the challenge and my experiences on the trails near Fort Ware stood me in good stead later on the Davie Trail.

The Store

Whenever I visited Charlie, we soon started discussing the price of flour, sugar, gas and other commodities. Discussing the availability of food was almost as common in Fort Ware as discussing the weather is down south. Maybe this was because so many of these northern people had suffered from a shortage of food supplies sometime during their lives. The older people in Fort Ware were very familiar with hunger. Out on their traplines, perhaps hampered by winter storms, they could run out of food while still a long way from home, as Tommy and Eva Poole were to relate to me later.

The "good old days" did not seem to have happened in Fort Ware, according to many people, and stories were often told of privation. At the turn of the twentieth century, a group of Sekani people had been found at Fort Grahame in a very bad way. Of the seven people in the group, five had died, "probably from starvation," and the survivors had been living on boiled flour. Food could be seen through the store windows but Fox, the store manager, was not at his post and the Sekani, it was reported, were too honest to break in to get the food. They were astounded when a white man broke open the door to gain access to the much-needed supplies.

In the winter of 1953, the people gathered together at Fort Ware, coming in from their camps, as they usually did, to receive trapline rations. For some reason, the Hudson's Bay post, after being open since 1927, had closed down and there was nothing available. Some people travelled down to Fort Grahame, but others stayed, risking starvation. At the same time, some Band members, called the Tsay Tuh and who lived at Caribou Hide, a small village northwest of Fort Ware, were even worse off. They were in danger of starving since there was no hope of their getting any provisions. The area around Caribou Hide was quite different from the land to the east, where there was an abundance of game. The empty Fort Ware store remained closed for three years.

As Samuel Black wrote in his journals after travelling through this area, there was a dearth of the animals that people relied on for food. Black, quoted by R.M. Patterson in his introduction to Black's diaries, suggests that Black's exploration occurred at a time of extended glaciation and maximum rain and cold, which would decrease animal activity in the area, something the Sekani tried to adapt to. Finally, after an outbreak of influenza that devastated the small group of people, they sought refuge at Metsantan, about 150 kilometres from Iskut, a Tahltan village. Then, because of continued privations, they moved over to Iskut, and Caribou Hide was abandoned, effectively separating the Tsay Tuh from some of their family members who had stayed in Fort Ware.

Ben Corke, a private trader, moved into Fort Ware in 1956, and the people were able to get supplies again. The supplies were very expensive, because they had to be driven by truck from Fort George to Summit Lake, then taken by river boat down the Crooked River to the Pack River, then against the current up the Parsnip and Finlay rivers. Ben Corke ran the store until 1963. At that point, Art Van Somer bought him out and ran the store until his sudden death in the early 1970s. His brother, Jim Van Somer, then took over until he retired in the 1980s. After the Van Somers retired, the Band ran the store until a comparatively new branch of the Hudson's Bay Company, called Northern Stores, was invited to manage it in the late 1990s. The store management had come full circle.

Before Northern Stores took over the management of the store in Fort Ware, it was a typical northern store. It was crowded with all the necessities of a northern life, and served as a meeting place for people who were waiting for a plane or just seeking a warm refuge where they could add to the usual village gossip. The building was painted a hideous blue, probably because the paint was available and cheap. It was managed by an eccentric,

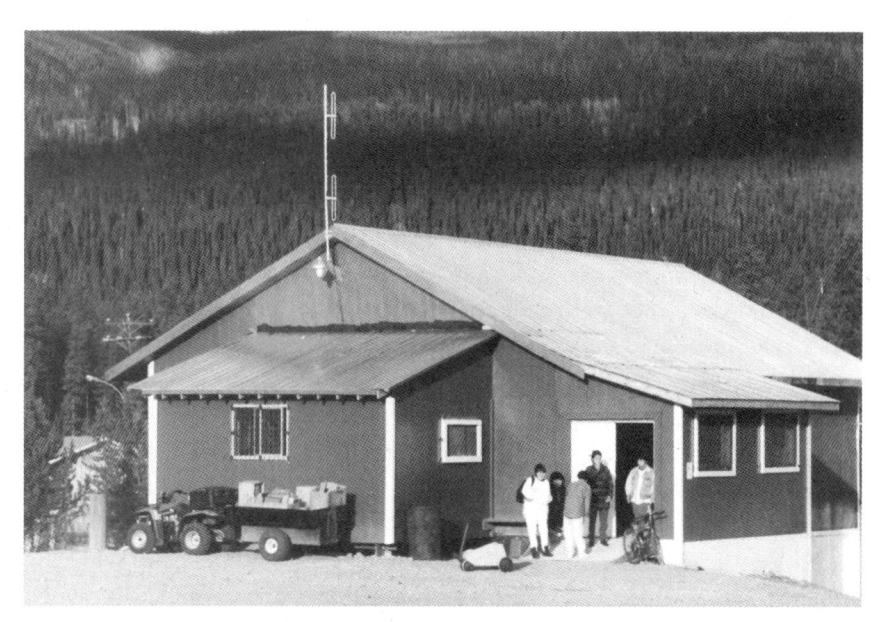

The old blue store in Fort Ware.

middle-aged Scot on behalf of the Band. His Scottish brogue could often be heard above the other chatter, giving orders to his staff. He was the epitome of the dour Scotsman, and yet apart from his gruff exterior, he was a generous man who loved a good joke. He ran the store on the lines of the old Hudson's Bay Company stores, because he had worked in their stores across the north before arriving in Fort Ware.

Rarely did you see the furs piled in the store that were such a familiar sight in other trading post stores. Although the Scottish store manager knew how to grade furs from his time working for the Hudson's Bay Company, he could only offer what the fur market dictated, and the trappers in Fort Ware had found that they could get more money for their furs if they sent them to the fur auctions. The problem with that option, however, was that they first had to find a way to get their furs out to the auction and then wait for the auction to take place before the money was received, and very few people wanted to wait for months.

Another option open to the trappers was to sell their furs to a buyer in Prince George, and so I became a courier of furs from Fort Ware. It was always interesting to take the furs into Black's Furs in Prince George, and go into the back room of the store and watch as the elderly storekeeper examined the furs, first shaking the fur out and then rubbing the palm of his hand over the hair so that he could assess the quality and checking to see that claws were on or off, as regulations dictated.

The Fort Ware store manager was always called "Colins," as in "Colin's store." At first I thought that it was a colloquial Sekani expression until I read about one of the Fort Grahame store managers who had the surname "Collins." Because he was a store manager, the Fort Grahame Collins would have been well known by the Sekani people. Collins normally stayed in Fort Grahame but he had once built a cabin at what became known as Collins Flat when he was stopped by ice on the river and had to protect all his stores. Storekeepers had the unenviable job of keeping the store financially viable, and Fort Ware's "Colins"—whose name actually was Colin Webster—was no exception. This meant that at times he had to cut off an individual's credit when a bill was long overdue and no attempt had been made to pay. Colin found that this was no way to win friends, but he would explain what the situation was and then make his decision. Colin's store, which was owned by the Band, made it possible for people to go out on their traplines by giving them credit, that is, an advance on their furs, just like in the old days. Some fur buyers (not connected to the Band in any way) would fly out to trapping cabins if they could land on a river or a lake, and pick up furs, paying cash. Store managers did not like this because the Native people might not be able to pay back their advance, but they would still expect one for the next season. Sometimes, if their credit was cut off, people would go and complain to Chief Emil McCook, but Emil would shrug and say he couldn't override the store manager's decision, and then he would tell people that they had to pay their bills if they wanted store credit.

What infuriated the store manager was when someone was at their credit limit and then received a large cheque for work or some other reason and would go out to the city and buy a big four-wheel bike or a new snowmobile, then still come and ask for more store credit. He once told one such person to go away and eat his new snowmobile if he was that desperate!

Although Colin had been a store manager for the Hudson's Bay Company in many places in the Northwest Territories and Nunavut before he came to Fort Ware, it seemed that he had found what he was looking for when he took over the Band-owned Fort Ware store. Once or twice he would get absolutely frustrated and quit on the spur of the moment, leaving the Band in a difficult situation. We would hire a replacement but after a few months the new manager would prove to be unsatisfactory for many and varied reasons and by then Colin was eager to come back to Fort Ware and we were quite pleased to have him back again. We were so desperate one spring that we chartered a plane to bring Colin back to British Columbia from Arctic Red River in the Northwest Territories in the middle of spring break-up. He arrived with the plane crammed full of his personal stuff, including his snowmobile.

A new store was built around the year 2000. It was designed to fit into the environment by using wood to a large extent, and when opened it was turned over—on Colin's recommendation—to Northern Stores to operate.

The Accident

While working for the Fort Ware Band, I came to know some people better than others, usually because I was involved in their lives in some way or another, often because of accident or illness. Such was the case with Christie Massettoe, the daughter of Daisy Massettoe and the granddaughter of Tommy and Eva Poole. After Christie was seriously injured by a falling tree, I spent many days and hours with the family and pieced together the details, using my knowledge of the family and their habits. The story shows the close family ties that exist in the Fort Ware community.

Tommy was an Elder who had a small house away from the main village on the bank of the Finlay River. He had his own generator for power and hauled his water from the Finlay River. He was a very independent man who travelled a long way up the Finlay to Bower Creek, where he hunted and trapped. He was a teetotaller, although his wife, Eva, was known to indulge occasionally. Tommy was a Band Councillor for a few years but his hearing deteriorated so that eventually he could not participate very well at meetings. Although his deafness was a hindrance in later years, he was extremely observant and would notice animals in the bush that other people missed entirely. I drove Tommy all over northern BC (along with other Band staff) and I helped him out when possible with clothes from the Salvation Army or Goodwill stores. I helped the family with shopping when they were in town, too. Tommy was an excellent river man and took me on several trips up the Finley River in his river boat.

Tommy had taken advantage of a sunny day to go and get a load of firewood. He had driven his quad motorbike to a likely-looking spot on the west side of the Finlay River. Some of his daughters and grandchildren had climbed on the bike to go along for a ride and to help carry the wood.

Tommy looked up at a dead pine tree and thought what a great piece of firewood it would make when it was cut up and split and ready for his woodstove. He noted how close it was to the trail and thought it would be easy to drop it where it could be cut up into stove lengths. Then his grandchildren would be quite happy to use his old quad bike to haul the logs back to his house on the bank of the Finlay River.

He took his chainsaw, filled it with gas and oil and walked over to the base of the tree. "You kids go back to the house and bring me a can of mixed gas. I'll need it to cut up this tree," he called out to the three girls who had come with him for the ride. He watched as they started back to the trail where the bike was parked. He felt for the can of Copenhagen chewing tobacco that was in his shirt pocket, took out a pinch and tucked it behind his lower lip, then called out, "Don't drive too fast, there's lots of time."

It took three pulls on the start rope before his chainsaw barked into life. After adjusting his hearing protectors, he started to make an undercut in the tree. He made another cut and the wedge piece soon shot out. He glanced up at the tree before placing the saw blade on the other side of the tree and started the last cut which would bring the tree down. The saw chain bit hungrily into the dry wood and soon the old tree started leaning, so Tommy quickly pulled out his saw, looking up at the tree as it started to fall. He glanced at where he wanted it to drop and was startled to see his eight-year-old granddaughter walking towards him, right in the path of the falling tree.

"NOOO! Christie, RUN!" Tommy shouted. Christie looked up and froze.

Tommy threw his chainsaw aside and ran towards Christie even as the tree hit the ground in a crash of broken branches. He arrived at a small depression at a point about eight feet from the top of the tree where it had broken off when it hit the ground. "Oh no, oh no, oh no," he muttered over and over, pulling the broken pieces of branches away from his granddaughter.

"Christie!" he cried out, "Christie!" In desperation he turned her over, immediately noticing a trickle of blood running out of the corner of her mouth, and then he saw that the top of her head was covered in blood too. With great relief, he saw that she was still breathing. He took his windbreaker off and wrapped her gently in it.

"Why did you come back?" he asked the unconscious girl. "I thought you'd all gone." He rocked backwards and forwards in his misery, his heart feeling cold. He looked forlornly down the trail for help, but all was quiet. He looked down at Christie, her long dark eyelashes covering eyes that had sparkled with excitement only moments before. Tommy couldn't prevent the tear that ran down his grizzled face and splashed on her cheek.

Tommy suddenly straightened up and listened intently, then with relief, he recognized the sound of his quad bike approaching. He waited until the engine had been turned off, then called out in a strained and cracked voice, "Over here!"

"Where?" his daughter Wendy called. Her voice came to him as though it was a million miles away.

"Here, by the tree!" Wendy ran up to where Tommy was kneeling by Christie.

"Oh, Dad, what happened?" Ashley had run up behind Wendy and now both girls bent and looked at Christie.

"Come on, let's get her to the clinic. Wendy, you grab her and I'll drive the bike." Ashley was already running down the trail to start the bike and turn it around. Wendy stooped down and gently took Christie in her arms and lifted her up with a strength she didn't know she possessed. She carefully stepped over the fallen tree and squeezed between it and an overgrown bush on the side of the road. When she reached the bike, she hoisted herself onto the rear carrier. Ashley drove the bike determinedly along the road to the clinic, a mile away.

Tommy sat still, unable to move in his shock and his grief. How could he have been so careless, he asked himself. Christie, she was so quiet, always wanting to help him. His thoughts went back to another occasion when he had sat by his second-oldest son, Andrew, and it seemed like another age. Andrew had been playing with his older brother out at their cabin up the river at Seven Mile Point, and the boys had sneaked a single shot .22-calibre rifle out of the cabin and were pretending to hunt. Tommy had heard a shot and then young Christopher had come running to him.

"Dad, come quick, Andrew got shot!" The memory of that moment ran like icicles through Tommy's veins. He had run to where Andrew lay, shot in the chest. He had picked him up and raced to his river boat moored on the riverbank. As he held his son, he had somehow managed to start the motor and as soon as Christopher had untied the boat, he raced it down the river to the village. Tears came to Tommy's eyes again as he remembered the nurse telling him that Andrew had probably died immediately and his race to the village had been in vain. Now here was quiet little Christie, and she was going to die too.

Community Health Nurse Judy Sandford was on one of her infrequent visits to Fort Ware when Wendy drove Christie to the clinic on her quad bike. Judy quickly evaluated the seriousness of Christie's injury. A Medivac plane was immediately summoned from Prince George but even so, it was several hours before Christie was transferred to Vancouver for cranial surgery.

The whole family travelled down to Vancouver with me. Several days after the surgery, Tommy was calling the unconscious Christie's name and felt her hand twitch in response. He was overwhelmed when he realized that she was not going to die, and I noticed a small tear run down his face as he bowed and whispered, "Thank you, Lord." In the next few days, Christie opened her eyes and slowly regained consciousness. When it was clear that she was recovering, the family returned with me to Fort Ware.

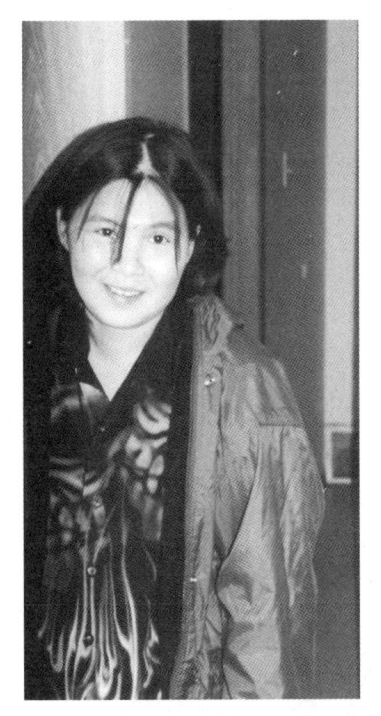

Christie Massettoe, the miracle girl.

Many weeks later, Northern Thunderbird Air arrived at a crowded landing strip in Fort Ware and disgorged its cargo. Then, at the top of the ramp, Christie appeared. "Look! It's the miracle girl!" someone shouted and Christie walked down the stairway and soon climbed into a waiting truck to sit by her grandpa. As the door was closed for her, I saw a small, shy smile creep across her face.

Serengeti of the North

Before the logging companies made inroads into Sekani country and before BC Hydro constructed the Peace River dam at Hudson's Hope to flood the valley, the Finlay River was prime moose habitat. A wildlife officer, Milt Warren, said during a survival course lecture to a group of government employees that the winding Finlay River with its gravel bars and willow islands had provided the shelter, food and protection from predators that the calving moose needed in the springtime. Now, with the changes to their habitat, the moose population had decreased. This decline was exacerbated by an influx of non-Native hunters who were always eager to drive to the end of newly developed logging roads in search of game. These were new areas for game management, but traditional hunting grounds for First Nations people.

The logged areas began to provide an abundance of new food, if not much protection, for the moose as the forest rejuvenated. The deer population increased but the increase was not noticeable to people from Fort Ware and Ingenika, who did not necessarily have trucks to hunt with and who had previously hunted along the Finlay River by river boat.

Grizzly bears and black bears were quite common, as were a variety of other animals. Wolves could often be heard howling in the distance and they had been seen on the perimeter of the village of Fort Ware, as had grizzly bears. Donny Van Somer shot a grizzly that walked through the village early one morning. Thankfully, it was hours before young children would have been walking to school.

On one occasion in the middle of winter, Emil McCook was driving his snowmobile along a trail not too far from the village when he looked down the trail and saw what he thought was a large wolf coming along the trail towards him. He stopped his machine and grabbed his rifle and took aim. The big black wolf—and Emil said that it looked *really* big—kept on coming towards him. This concerned him quite a bit, so he shot it. After carefully walking up to it with his rifle held ready, he saw that it wasn't a wolf at all but a big black bear! He told me that bears did not come out of hibernation for another two months so he concluded that the bear had been disturbed by something and had walked down the trail to keep out of the deep snow. He skinned out the bear, salted the hide, then took the meat home and put it and the hide in his freezer. Later on, he asked me if I would like to have the hide because he needed the freezer space. So if you ever visit my house you will see the black bear, now a rug, in front of the fireplace.

The logging road provided some excellent opportunities to see wild animals and birds. Never before, or since, have I seen such a number and variety of animals in the wild. I always carried my camera with me, but the animals were reluctant to wait around to be photographed while I stopped my truck and grabbed my camera, so most of the time I had to be content with exciting memories.

One of the most memorable trips that I made to Fort Ware on the Finlay Main logging road was on May 1, 2001. The road was quiet, the sun was shining, and I was making a leisurely trip up to the village when I saw an incredible number of wild animals: seven bears and two cubs, one wolf, one coyote, ten moose, fourteen deer, and a whole herd of elk. This was, of course, over the course of six or seven hours of driving on an isolated logging road. On my return trip five days later, I saw one coyote, a grizzly bear, a beaver crossing the road, six bears and two cubs, one moose, one elk and a crossfox (a fox with a coat of different colours, some black, white and red). I couldn't have done better visiting a city zoo.

One early morning, I was driving south from Fort Ware on a cold winter's morning when coming around a sharp bend in the road I saw five jet-black wolves on the road. Within seconds they had looked up, startled, I thought, and then without a glance back at me they jumped over the snowbank and ran up a half-frozen creek.

Twice I have encountered a family of lynx on the road. The first time there were two adults with four half-grown kittens. The adults went to one side of the road and the kittens to the other. They waited until I had passed and then were reunited. A curious sighting was of five lynx gathered in the middle of the road. These normally shy cats must have had something on their minds, perhaps breeding, because only after I honked my horn did they reluctantly climb on to the snowbank and sidle over the side.

Another time in the late afternoon, I came over a hill and saw a strange apparition running with a peculiar gait up the road in front of me. It almost looked like it was running sideways. I drove up close to try to identify it and saw that it had a light diamond pattern on his otherwise dark brown back. I was following a seldom-seen wolverine. I slowed down but suddenly he reversed his direction and came right at me. With a rumble, it went under the centre of the truck and I stopped immediately. Through the rear view mirror I could see it lying in the road. I got out to look closely and came to within a metre of it when tough old Mr. Wolverine jumped up, shook himself and high-tailed it down the road, again with his peculiar gait. Apparently he had not broken any bones and I was glad that he had run off in the direction opposite to where I was standing. Wolverines are one of the fiercest animals and will rob food from even the bigger carnivores.

Cow moose, with or without calves, moose with huge antlers, deer, elk and bears were all common on the Finlay Road. Late one night when I was heading to Fort Ware in my truck along with Emil and Craig McCook, Hazel Boya's brother, we heard someone on the road radio channel asking for help because he had hit a moose, killing it, and now the truck was hung up over the moose carcass. The accident had happened about ten kilometres north of where we were and we arrived at the scene in a very short time. The driver was unhurt and his large pickup truck had not suffered any damage that we could see, but his reinforced bumper had killed the moose and then the high-centred truck had ridden up on the animal.

The only implement that we had between us was a small penknife Craig had. He started to cut the moose's head off, but there was so much road grit in the animal's hair that he had to keep sharpening his knife on a stone. Emil was trying to help, but he had been drinking earlier in the evening and he was still "a bit dizzy," he said. Covered in mud and blood they managed to cut off the moose's head, which they threw into the back of my pickup truck. (They wanted the nose and the tongue, both considered delicacies.) We managed to pull the vehicle off the moose with my tow rope,

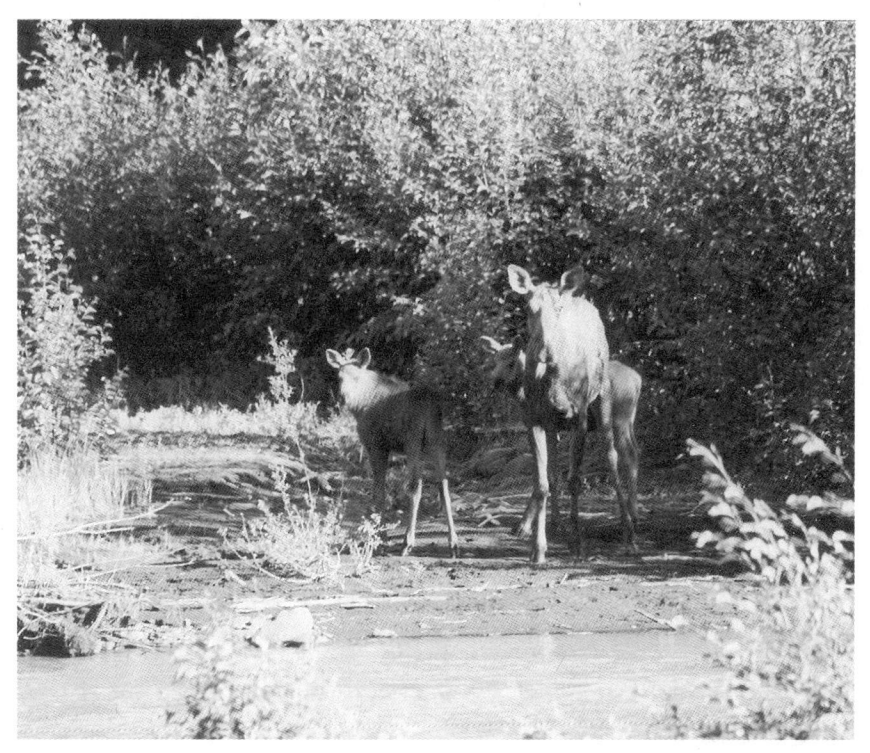

The "Serengeti of the North" is home to many animals, including this moose and her twin calves.

but the moose was so mangled that neither Emil or Craig wanted it for meat, especially if they had to cut it up with a penknife. Over an hour later we continued on our way, my truck now reeking of sweat, blood and mud—but at least the cool night air had sobered up Emil.

Early one springtime when I was driving up to Fort Ware, I had just stopped to take a photograph of a bald eagle in a tree by the side of the road when I saw a black object high in a cottonwood tree, then I saw two very small black objects in another tree. A mother black bear with two cubs! Thinking that I had a good photo op, I grabbed my camera, climbed out of the pickup and walked to the side of the road. Mamma black bear was not having any of this and she came down her tree almost as fast as I ran back to my truck and slammed the door.

I think that the most unusual and interesting animal I saw was a cougar that crossed the road in front of me when I was driving south with old Tommy Poole. Tommy said it was obvious that the deer numbers were increasing if a cougar had come that far north because they had not been sighted in the area before.

One unfortunate thing that I did was stop on the road to peer at a small furry creature coming up the snowy road. It did not move to the right or the left but kept coming right past the truck. Out of curiosity I backed up so that I could find out what it was. I found out sure enough because when I backed up, I squashed the poor little muskrat flat under a tire. There wasn't a pond or swamp anywhere near so I could not think what it was doing cruising up the road.

On another occasion, driving south with two young Sekani men from Fort Ware, I was again involved in a moose incident. A call came over the road radio channel from a man who had hit a moose.

"I just ran into a moose at kilometre 165 and the moose is still alive. Has anyone got a gun?" he said.

No one answered on the radio. I radioed to the caller: "We don't have a gun, but I've got two Fort Ware guys with me and they'll know what to do."

I turned to one of the men with me. "You guys will know what to do without a gun, won't you?" I asked confidently.

"I've only killed a moose with a gun," he replied. "Those things can kick, you know." The other young fellow just nodded.

Twenty minutes later, on a straight stretch of road, we saw the pickup truck pulled over to the side of the road against a snowbank. On the other side of the road lay the moose, still struggling to get up, but one front and one back leg were obviously broken in several places. In its struggles, the animal had pushed itself up against the snowbank opposite the truck.

"Here's my sheath knife. It should do the job," I offered hopefully.

"There's no way I'm going near it!" the younger man said. I realized that these fellows were not much more than teenagers and had not been out in the bush very much. Well, we couldn't leave the moose as it was, so I went over to look at it with the other truck driver.

The moose looked at me and kicked ineffectually and I said that I would try to kill it with my knife. An old Gwich'in man had shown me how to dispatch wounded caribou when I lived in the Northwest Territories. He said that you had to cut their spinal cord just where the skull sits on the spine. He said this was so the animal would die fast, he would save a rifle shell and the meat would not be spoiled. I wasn't worried about saving a gun shell or spoiling the meat but I wanted it to die quickly for the moose's sake, and mine. I knew that a kick from a full-grown moose could be lethal so I approached the animal from the frozen snowbank so that I could come up from behind him.

There is something very uncomfortable about sticking a knife into something alive, especially when it is watching you with what seemed to be very big and belligerent eyes. I kneeled, estimated where I should stab, took a deep breath and steeled myself. I grasped the knife handle firmly and thrust it into the back of the animal's neck.

It struck a bone. I jumped back quickly as the moose struggled and kicked before it quietened again. I looked at the moose and it looked back at me with a large staring eye. I reassessed the back of the neck, my fingers probing the base of the skull. Ah, there, I could feel a soft spot. I placed the point of the knife on the spot and pushed the knife in with all my might. The moose's legs stiffened and its body quivered, about the same reaction as mine, but the knife had done the job and the moose was dead.

Now the two young men seemed to be galvanized into action.

"C'mon, we have to cover up the moose now it's dead!"

"Why?"

"The old people say that something bad will happen if we don't cover it after it's been killed."

"Okay, you go ahead. There's a shovel in the back of my truck."

The other driver and I walked over to my truck and we shared a cup of coffee from my Thermos while the boys tried shovelling the hard-packed snow over the moose. I thought that the wolves would soon be along and they would clean it up, and when I came back that way a few days later all that was left was moose hair strewn over the road and over the snowbank.

The Road, the Lake, and the Booze

In the mid-1990s, the logging road was pushed north to within fifteen kilometres of Fort Ware. There it was to turn east towards the Finlay River, where a winter bridge that would cross over to Buffalo Head logging camp was planned. When we saw that there were no plans to bring it to the village, representations were made to the logging contractor and by reminding them that they were in Fort Ware territory, a reasonable price was negotiated to have the road built right to the Finlay River opposite the village.

The road was a mixed blessing because now freight for the village could be trucked from Prince George right to Fort Ware—except the road stopped on the opposite side of the river. The truck had to be unloaded by hand, the freight carried to a river boat and loaded, floated over to the other side, and then unloaded on the shore and driven up to the store or the school by several quad bikes. Still labour-intensive!

When the wind blew up Williston Lake from the south, whipping up ocean-sized waves, logging debris loosened from the bottom of the lake floated to the surface where it blocked the mouth of the Finlay River. This was always treacherous and sometimes impossible to navigate through. BC

The Road, the Lake, and the Booze   67

Hydro occasionally supplied a small tug to force a way through the logs so that the supply boats could get through. I once sent my truck down the lake on a small barge late in the fall. When it arrived in Mackenzie, it was entirely covered with over eight centimetres of hard ice after high waves had crashed over the barge and immediately frozen on the cold vehicle.

The only advantage of the lake was that it flooded Deserters' Canyon where the Finlay River had surged through. In times past, boatmen would have to line or winch their boats to the top end of the canyon, or make several trips with reduced loads. However, this advantage was negated by the debris.

Deserters' Canyon had been named by Samuel Black after he had passed that way on his exploration of the Finlay River. On May 27, 1824, two of his party, Jean Marie Bouche and Louis Ossin, two of his "half breed voyageurs," deserted at this critical point on the river when they were portaging their canoe and equipment round this treacherous canyon. They left unexpectedly and unannounced but well supplied with both company and private property. However, they turned themselves in at the Hudson's Bay Company post at Ile-à-la-Crosse, where they were punished—although the punishment was said to be less than they would have experienced had they continued travelling with Samuel Black.

Because there was no viable alternative for freighting fuel oil to the village, it was flown in by Northern Thunderbird Air from an airstrip that had been constructed at the mouth of the Ingenika River where the Forestry Department had a fire suppression crew and a fire retardant tanker base. There was also a group of First Nations people who lived close to the airstrip, who were victims of high-handed government policy-makers. Before the Williston dam had been built, these people had lived at Fort Grahame on the lower reaches of the Finlay River. In 1914, five federal commissioners had visited and set aside eight hundred acres for the Sekani people at Fort Grahame. In spite of this, the government decided to relocate the Band, then called the Ingenika Band, to a specially created reserve on the left bank of the Parsnip River so that flooding of the valley could commence. It seemed that there was a complete lack of understanding by the bureaucracy about the Sekani way of life when they were settled many miles away from their traplines and traditional hunting areas. The graveyard at Fort Grahame was flooded as were the old buildings, cabins and the log Hudson's Bay Company store and church.

The new reserve was located on a paved road that led to Mackenzie. It had modern new houses, complete with a water system and hydro power to each house, but the relocation turned into a disaster. People now had easy access to liquor and vented their anger and frustrations with the government by overindulging, with the result that fights and wife and child abuse became common. A small group of Sekani could stand the situation no longer and, under the leadership of Gordon Pierre, they moved to Ingenika Point, close to where the airstrip had been made for the Forest Service. The Department of Indian Affairs refused to give these renegade Sekani any housing material because they were considered squatters, so these resilient people built small log houses and purchased what they needed whenever they could afford it. By trapping and hunting, these few people were successful in providing for their families, and Harvey Simms, who had a small store at the Point, bought their furs and provided groceries. There was no alcohol in the new village and as their success became known, more and more of the Parsnip Reserve people made their way back until eventually the government-sanctioned Reserve on the Parsnip River was abandoned. Slowly over the ensuing years it reverted to nature, with trees and shrubs filling in the roads. The Forest Service took over the area again and it became part of a cutblock and the remaining trees were cut down.

Eventually, after many years of fighting, the Band, now called the Tse Keh Neh, were able to negotiate a land claims agreement using the powerful legal weight of Eddie John, a First Nations lawyer and Tribal Chief from Tache Reserve on Stewart Lake. Their new village now lies close to the mouth of the Finlay River. From there, the Elders can look south down Williston Lake with its 1,770-kilometre shoreline that surrounds their drowned homes.

A Beech 18 aircraft was fitted with a large bladder that could be filled with fuel oil at Ingenika, and then flown to Fort Ware. There it was piped to holding tanks near the school. Few accidents occurred transporting fuel this way. One did occur when the pilot, who had made numerous fifteen-minute flights between Ingenika and Fort Ware, came in for a landing and neglected to lower the Beechcraft's wheels. That ended the fuel haul for quite a while.

A second accident occurred when a side feeder line was inadvertently left open in Fort Ware. This feeder pipe had been used for pumping the fuel oil to the school from the river when it had been brought up by boat. Later, when the extension pipe from the airport was attached, the valve for the pipe that went to the river was inadvertently opened and the oil ran into the river. This upset a lot of people concerned with the environment as well as the Department of Indian Affairs, which had purchased the oil.

Fortunately though, we never observed any dead fish or any other untoward effects from this spill.

One of the negative effects of the road was the easy access for bootleggers to bring alcohol into Fort Ware. The Reserve had been designated as "dry" by the Chief and Council, that is, no alcohol was supposed to be allowed on Native land, not even homebrew, and the police had the authority to confiscate liquor from vehicles headed to Fort Ware or any containers of liquor that were found during routine patrols of the village. One of the problems with enforcing this was that the police, who had a new detachment at Ingenika, only came to Fort Ware occasionally unless there was a problem that they had to investigate.

Before the road was built, people had made homebrew to quench their thirst, and a small quantity of hard liquor was brought in by some individuals and sold at very inflated prices. With road access, some entrepreneurs began bringing in pickup trucks loaded with alcohol that they continued to sell at these inflated prices, some bottles of whiskey costing a hundred dollars. To me, this seemed most unfair because the effect of this liquor was much worse than that of homebrew and some people were spending what little money they had on something that increased the social ills of the village and had no benefits at all for the residents. As usual, it was the children who suffered. If I happened to be in Fort Ware when a large amount of alcohol was seized, I was asked by the visiting RCMP corporal to witness the destruction of the contents and it always saddened me to see hundreds of dollars wasted by people who had bought the alcohol with their meagre funds only to lose their money in this way. I was asked to witness the destruction so that the RCMP officers could not be accused of keeping it for themselves.

Circuit Court

Until the 1980s, whenever residents of Fort Ware were called on to attend court, the accused and the witnesses had to make their own way to Mackenzie, where the court was held, unless the accused was in custody. If they were just summoned to appear, they would travel to Mackenzie by river boat or the lucky ones would hitch a ride on someone's chartered plane. At Mackenzie, they just camped in the bush while they waited to be called to the courthouse by their lawyers. If the accused was fortunate and held in the RCMP cells, he had a comparatively warm and comfortable bed and three meals a day. The witnesses and even the victims in these cases spent their time in the only warm place that would accept them, the pub, and by the time they were needed in the court, some of them found themselves too drunk to be of any use in the proceedings and some ended up being charged for being intoxicated in a public place. The whole thing became one vicious circle and finally the courts, the lawyers and the judge realized that this was causing more problems than it was trying to solve.

In the 1940s, only serious cases found their way to court and, because travelling was so difficult, nothing happened in a hurry. A book entitled *Policing A Pioneer Province, 1858–1950* by Lynne Stonier-Newman describes the time when British Columbia had its own provincial police force. The book includes a description of an investigation of a murder in Fort Ware, when Tommy Poole's father, Steven Poole, murdered his wife.

On January 11th 1943 word was received from Fort Ware on the Upper Finlay River that an Indian woman had died under circumstances pointing to murder. The only way of reaching Fort Ware at that time of the year was by plane and as the weather was bad Sergeant Clark of Prince George was unable to reach Fort Ware until January 30th.

On arrival the sergeant learned that on January 8th, Margaret Poole had gone to visit with a native trapper and his wife who lived a distance down the river. Her husband, Steven Poole, a non-native, joined them for supper, dancing and drinking. About 9 pm, the couple left to return to their own cabin, followed by Tommy, their ten year old son. When the sergeant questioned him, Tommy said that his father had started to beat his mother with a rifle butt, and when he tried to interfere he was knocked out of the way. Poole then removed most of his wife's clothing, making it appear that she had frozen to death. That evidence confirmed the message a trapper had sent to the police after seeing Margaret's battered body two days later.

As the weather was closing in fast, Clark decided to go back out on the plane to bring in a magistrate and coroner. He left behind a special constable, directing him to try and locate Poole out on his trap-line. Clark expected to fly back in the next day. However on the return trip when the plane landed for fuel at Findlay Forks [sic], a cylinder cracked, stranding the group there until a replacement part arrived on February 15th. Then the weather closed down and it was not until March 2nd that [the group] reached Fort Ware. Captain Dawson performed an autopsy on Margaret Poole's exhumed body and Coroner Harris held an inquest. Poole was charged with the murder of his wife and committed for trial.

One of the group later added to the official report recalling that it had been a memorable trip. It had been almost midnight when, after the autopsy, the murdered woman was returned to her grave. The wind and the wolves howled as they carried the thawed body back up the hill through the blizzard, scraped snow out of the hole dynamited for her first burial, and placed her in it again. Someone said a few words then they hurried back to the cabin and spent the night in crowded discomfort. The next day, the weather closing in fast, they had all squeezed aboard the plane for the trip out: two policemen, the prisoner and his two children, the coroner, the doctor and the Indian agent. They had to sit with arms and legs entangled in order to fit everyone on board—which became unpleasant when the children got airsick. "One just had to sit there and get splashed and try not to vomit oneself. It was a rough trip."

Circuit court these days is very different from that "rough trip" in 1943. Now the lawyers, social workers, court reporters and the judge travel to Fort Ware by turbo prop plane and hold court in the Fort Ware Community Hall on a quarterly basis. The court usually lasts for two or three days and is conducted like any southern court, with stenographers, recordings and protocols all in place. The judge sits at a table in front of the community hall stage. The court stenographers sit to his or her left with their bank of recorders in front of them and the microphone wires leading off in every direction. As is usual in a court, the lawyers sit at several tables facing the judge and always rise to address him or her.

Whenever the lawyers or other counsel or even the RCMP enter the main room, they always bow towards the judge. Meanwhile, members of the audience enter and leave the room at will without following any such etiquette and dozens of curious people congregate in the hallway and peer through the windows into the courtroom. Sometimes there appears to be utter confusion as individuals are called and, in some court sessions, witnesses who were bored or tired went home for a while. If this happened, another case would be called and chances are that if this was their first appearance it would be held over until the next court session in three or four months' time. There are one or two trials per session. These may last all day with breaks for some other minor cases. Courts were interesting to observe but I couldn't help feeling that there should be a more organized way of doing things.

When the court first came to Fort Ware, the Band was given the chance to supply the food and meals for the court party and for a couple of people to earn a few dollars as cooks. Everything went well at first, then one time the cook came to me in the court and said that everything was ready in the log building where the court party were all staying, the table was laid and the food set out. I went down to the cabin just before court ended to check things out and noticed that the door was open. I went in and, to my horror, I saw three large scruffy dogs actually standing on the table eating the food. Getting some help, we quickly cleaned things up and managed to salvage some food. It was one of those times when the best-laid plans (and tables) went almost completely to the dogs!

The final straw came when on another court day, the cook came to the cabin in a mildly intoxicated state and considering who the guests were, she was not allowed to continue. The court party was fed with half-thawed, half-frozen lasagna and a hurriedly prepared salad and garlic toast. In despair, I told the judge that it was just too difficult for us to manage, meaning that it was too difficult for me to manage, and afterwards the court administrator in Prince George contracted with a professional cook who brought in all the supplies and managed the whole thing. It took a weight off my shoulders and the advantage was that I was always invited to supper with the court party. To make things more comfortable for the visitors, one of the newer houses in the village was designated as a visitors' residence. It happened to have white siding and before long everyone referred to it as the "White House." When the court party was in the village, the house was quite crowded but everyone always got on very well and there were no problems.

It took me a while to adjust to seeing the court party relaxing and being informal in the residence, the defence counsel and the prosecution lawyers usually talking about other legal cases, while the judge listened in and sometimes commented. In the court when one side or the other would refer to "my friend," indicating the opposing counsel, it made me think that he would really like to say "this idiot here"! Of course they were all friends and the judge would sometimes chastise one of the lawyers if they got too "uppity." I wondered if their acting was to impress their clients, each other or the judge. The judge did not take any sides and kept everything moving from one case to the next. Most of the members of the RCMP from the Tseh Keh detachment were present, usually as witnesses, but I suspect that they were there to ensure the safety of the court party too. A couple of sheriffs would attend if there was someone in custody or if it were anticipated that someone soon would be.

Court was usually very interesting and I was appointed by Chief Emil McCook to speak on behalf of Fort Ware Council and various Band members. With social services cases, I was asked if I would like to cross-examine witnesses. Quite a change from Band administration and nursing responsibilities.

One time I was driving out from Fort Ware after court when the weather had closed in and the planes stopped flying. I stopped at Tseh Keh village with a message for a member of the court party and found that everyone was stranded there. One of the lawyers asked if he and the judge could ride out with me and though I explained that the crew cab truck was full of supplies, they said that they would still like to squeeze in. The back of the truck was loaded with all sorts of equipment and at the top of the pile I had fastened the court cook's boxes of pans and cooking utensils, which I was taking out for him. Everything went fine until at about ten-thirty at night, I hit a huge pothole and my carefully packed truck started scattering the cook's supplies along the road. I stopped, and with the aid of a flashlight, started picking up spatulas, bowls, carving knives and other cooking paraphernalia. Soon I was joined by the lawyer and the judge and we hunted through the dust and gravel of the road picking up supplies, then sweaty and dusty, we fastened everything back on the truck and continued on our way. By two o'clock in the morning, I was very tired and would normally have pulled over and had a sleep, but this time the lawyer offered to drive the truck. He was not familiar with the road but we pulled into Prince George safely just before dawn. No one from the court party ever asked me for a ride after that!

Not all the offenses that occurred in Fort Ware ended up in court; in fact, some were not even reported to the police. Early one cold and snowy morning, I was called to a house where a middle-aged man was said to have fallen on a knife. His wife asked me to take a look at him to see if his injury was serious. Serious? He was lying on a couch clutching his abdomen when I entered the living room. There was the unmistakable odour of alcohol. "What happened?" I asked.

"I was going downstairs and tripped and fell on my knife."

"At six o'clock in the morning?"

"I was going to cut some meat."

I wasn't a policeman but it sometimes helps to know the circumstances of an accident when trying to assess the severity of an injury. I moved his hands where he was holding them protectively against his lower abdomen. A bulge of intestine was poking through a five-centimetre cut in the abdominal wall.

"You're going to need some surgery for this. How long ago did it happen?" I looked at the dried and caked blood around the wound, which looked as though it had been there for hours.

"It just happened," he said, without looking at me.

"I'm going to phone a doctor," I said, and his wife showed me where the phone was. Fortunately there was a doctor visiting at Tseh Keh who was planning on leaving the village later in the morning to fly back to Prince George and I was able to reach him at the village health centre.

"Bring him down here right away and I'll see what I can do." It was the obvious answer.

I hurried to the local clinic and the community health worker gave me some gauze and a bottle of saline solution and then I hurried back to the patient's house. It took a few minutes to clean around the wound and to wrap some saline-soaked gauze around the intestine and tape a dressing over it. Then I half-carried him down to my truck, put a seat belt on him and away we drove.

Using my two-way road radio, I spoke into the microphone: "This is a pickup truck heading south from Fort Ware with a medical emergency! I will have my four-way hazard light on." I stood hard on the gas pedal, almost sending the truck into a spin on an icy corner so I reminded myself to take it easy or else there would be two patients. I passed an oncoming empty logging truck that flew by me sending a shower of snow and gravel into my windshield. The driver had not heard my radio call or didn't care.

I arrived at the Tseh Keh clinic and the nurse there helped me carry the patient into the examining room where the doctor was waiting. He examined the wound and casually said, "Well, we can't do anything with this here. We'll leave the dressing that Keith put on and send him to Prince George. The plane should be here in about an hour."

I thought my part in this little episode was now over but the nurse asked me to stay and help get the patient to the plane at the airstrip, which was about five kilometres north of the village. Over a cup of coffee in the clinic, the doctor said that the wound looked very much like a stab wound and not like a wound that would have been sustained by someone falling down the stairs onto a knife. He said that they would have to explore the wound in the operating room to make sure that no part of the intestine itself had been cut.

I drove the patient and the doctor to the airplane when it arrived and waited for the plane to leave before I drove back up to Fort Ware, my morning used up as an ambulance driver, something else to add to my resume. I do not think that the RCMP were involved at all, so whether there had been a drunken fight the night before was anyone's guess, but no one was admitting to anything.

Although there has never been a manned RCMP detachment in Fort Ware, the police tried to visit routinely. In 2011, a detachment was being constructed by the Band in the village, maybe with the hope that "if they build it, they will come." In spite of its isolation, services to Fort Ware are slowly improving and the new RCMP detachment is the latest move forward, although it has taken nearly a hundred years to get this far.

When they were forging their way to the gold fields to try to bring law and order to the Yukon, the Royal Northwest Mounted Police were kept busy making a trail from Edmonton and through the Peace River area, because they were expecting that the Klondikers would go north en masse through the Rocky Mountain Trench, which seemed to travel straight to the gold fields in the Yukon. The job was given to Inspector Moodie, who took with him four constables and an Iroquois guide. After setting out from Edmonton in September 1897, they finally arrived at the Finlay River on January 16. They travelled for two more days before reaching Fort Grahame. Then after travelling many more miles to replenish their supplies, they left Fort Grahame in July and carried on up the Finlay River to the point where it turns west. They followed the Fox River north on the Davie Trail, over Sifton Pass—which Inspector Moodie named after Clifford Sifton, a federal cabinet minister, in 1898.

In 1905, the RNWMP "big brass" set out again from Edmonton to make a trail from the Peace River, heading west to the Finlay River. Then they were to try and make a trail over the mountains, still heading west. Superintendent Constantine and Inspector Richards, along with six officers and twenty-two constables, were confronted by cold weather and deep snow but an advance party arrived at Fort Grahame, where they spent the winter before continuing west. They finally did reach the Telegraph Trail but it was useless because Klondikers were in a hurry to go north, not west, and before long the trail had reverted to nature. An area south of Fort Ware where the police camped and wintered their horses is still called "Police Meadows." It is now an Indian Reserve under the jurisdiction of the Tse Keh Dena.

Mapping the Davie Trail

The Davie Trail originally started in northern British Columbia at Finlay Forks, located at the junction of the Finlay and Parsnip rivers. In 1867, the trailhead was moved when the Hudson's Bay Company opened a post a few kilometres farther south at the junction of the Finlay and the Peace rivers. This post was named Fort Grahame, after James Grahame, a senior Hudson's Bay Company official.

When the southern part of the Rocky Mountain Trench was flooded by BC Hydro between 1960 and 1970, the Finlay, Nation, Crooked and Parsnip rivers now all emptied into the newly formed Williston Lake, from which the Peace River starts its tortuous journey on its way to the Beaufort Sea hundreds of miles to the north. After the valley was flooded, trails, cabins and cultural sites disappeared along with a part of the Davie Trail, so that now the trail starts, or ends, at Fort Ware, eighty kilometres north of Williston Lake.

The instigator of a practical down-to-earth research project to assert the land claims to the Davie Trail by the Kaska people was the inimitable Charlie Boya. Charlie and his wife, Hazel, had a vested interest in the trail because of their trapline and cabin at Terminus Mountain. They worried that if the trail was unused, it would disappear into the bush unless animals kept parts of it open as they wandered to and from their grazing or breeding areas. Worse still was the possibility that the government could lay claim to the area and open it up to exploitation by industrialists.

It is almost impossible to grasp the enormity of the isolated area through which the Davie Trail runs. The trail winds past and through the Muskwa-Kechika Management area, a protected area of 6.4 million hectares (15 million acres)—roughly the size of Ireland and almost as large as the American state of Maine. At the southern end of the trail, near Fort Ware, it runs close to Kwadacha Provincial Park and Northern Rockies Provincial Park, which together cover 665,707 hectares, or 1,644,939 acres of land.

In conversation with Elders in the Fort Ware community, the words "tradition" and "trail" invariably came up when the conversation turned to the land north of Fort Ware. The Elders wanted the younger people to be aware of the trail because it was their heritage, their history, the story of their lives. Knowledge of the trail was something they felt had to be handed down from generation to generation if they were to survive as a nation.

Charlie was aware of the general lack of use of the trail by First Nations people. Although he regularly travelled perhaps a hundred kilometres north in the winter when he did some trapping or moose hunting, he knew that no travellers had walked the entire Davie Trail since he had been a young boy. As a child, he had lived on a section of the trail with his father, Louis Boya. Louis had trapped the whole northern part of the territory from Lower Post, but few people had been on those traplines since Louis had retired. Charlie felt that the Kaska land claims negotiators were going to be on thin ice claiming frequent use of the land along the trail.

Lobbying for money to pay for a group of Kaska people to go up or down the trail (Charlie didn't mind which), he, along with Eric Gunderson from the Northwest Environmental Group in Williams Lake, finally convinced the Kaska Tribal Council to provide some funding in the late 1990s to clear a few kilometres of trail and to plot the whole length of it on a map. The Tribal Council contracted with Charlie to act as a guide so that some of the trail's physical characteristics would be documented to help in their land claims.

Charlie Boya had hoped that the trail-cutting would begin at Fort Ware, but for political and funding reasons the Kaska Tribal Council decided to start the project at Watson Lake. The northern portion of the Davie Trail is virtually unknown today to most of the Sekani people of Fort Ware, but even those people with Kaska lineage living in Lower Post and Watson Lake did not know many of the trail details. Charlie was the only person who was familiar with the trail from Fort Ware to Terminus Mountain. In the northern areas that were unfamiliar, even though he had been on the northern section as a boy, he said that he could find his way, using his "bush know how."

Charlie, cautious as ever, needed someone at the Band's administrative level to help him out with logistics—preferably someone on the Band payroll so that there would not be too much demand on the money allotted by the Kaska Council and there would be sufficient money for himself and the other members of the team. That someone turned out to be me.

I spent many evenings with Charlie and Hazel, listening to them tell stories about life at their cabin on the Kechika River and their adventures as they travelled up and down the Davie Trail. The more I heard of the trail, the more I thought that it would be an amazing wilderness experience to walk its length, an opportunity to see wild animals in their natural unspoiled environment—but it was nothing but a dream until Charlie and Hazel invited me to join them. Charlie and Hazel gave me the invitation to go with them one evening when we were sitting in their house talking about the trail. They said that they were going to hike down the 460-kilometre Davie Trail from Lower Post to Fort Ware, and would I like to go with them?

To be able to live and travel with people who really knew the country and whose ancestors had travelled the trails for centuries was a gift indeed. Ever since I had first flown over the area, I had thought about the people who lived in the cabins below me and what their lives were like, and now I would be able to learn first-hand by experiencing something of it.

Emil McCook, the Chief and the person to whom I was answerable, gave me his enthusiastic approval to go on the trek, happy that a non-Native employee wanted to see the land with which he himself felt a close affinity. Emil had always encouraged me to explore the land, and constantly said, "Don't be in a rush, Keith. Take your time to smell the roses." Rather subtly, he also reminded me of an important Band Council meeting coming up concerning a multi-million-dollar new school and which he asked me to attend as soon as I expected to get back from hiking the trail. The timing was going to be tight.

I had no qualms about being able to make the hike although some friends and family jokingly questioned whether they would ever see me again. I had to acknowledge that I was not exactly in the prime of life, just coming up to my sixtieth birthday. But my philosophy has always been that you are as old as you feel and that age is purely a state of mind—although

80   Tse-loh-ne

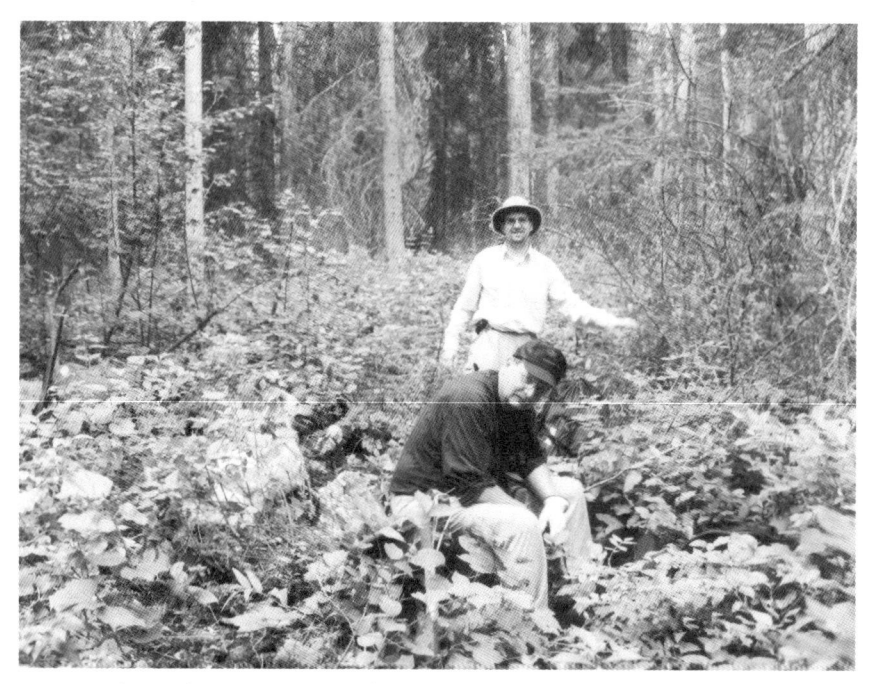

In many places, the Aatse Davie Trail is overgrown and tangled.

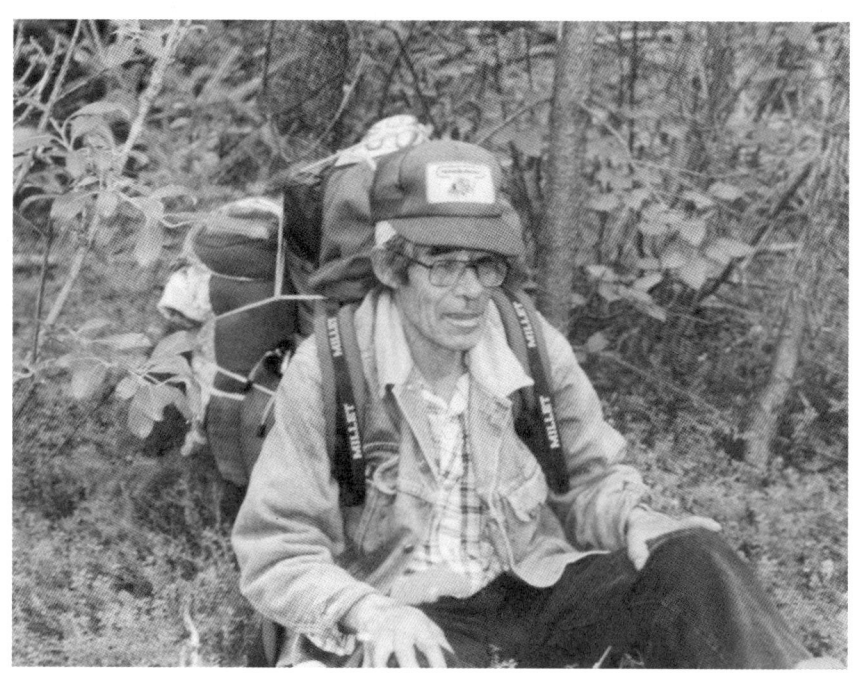

Antoine Charlie is ready for the trail.

there were times at the end of a hard day's hike when I began to wonder if I would ever see my next birthday!

A trail is defined as "a rough, ill-defined road in wild country." The Davie Trail is probably the longest "ill-defined road" in all of northern British Columbia. Although to most people it was nothing but a track through the bush, to people with imagination and who had taken the time to find out the history of the trail, it was like having the pages of a book turned for you as you walked by rivers and mountains and old cabins and heard of the trials and pleasures that the Native people experienced as they travelled up and down the trail. I wanted to have the total experience of the old-timers who had walked this and other trails but in reality the total experience could not be achieved because clothing and equipment are now far superior to that available to the old-timers.

Our plan was to spend two to three weeks on the northern section of the trail, with four pack dogs to help carry the supplies. For this first part of the trip south from the Dease River, close to Lower Post, which is the start of the Davie Trail, Charlie Boya had recruited a bush-wise couple from Fort Ware to be the camp organizers and cook. When I was told that the couple was Antoine and Annie Charlie, I was a bit surprised. Although I had previously met the couple, I didn't know them very well, but I did know that they spent most of their time out in the bush at one of their cabins. I also knew that they partied quite extensively and I didn't want to be involved with something that could hinder the "expedition" and at the same time make me feel very uncomfortable. Charlie Boya was convinced that the couple would work hard and not cause any problems but I knew that hard work or specific knowledge did not always guarantee that there would not be any problems.

A person that I knew well and who had worked for the Band had been such a man and his demise had been caused by binge drinking. Buzz Van Somer, Jim's son, was the Band's maintenance person. He could drive anything—backhoes, graders, heavy-duty trucks with air brakes, even Caterpillar tractors. He had a fair knowledge of plumbing and building and he could put his hand to almost anything but, "I don't do electricity," he once told me. Buzz worked hard, and I have known him to work along with contractors on emergency repairs from six in the morning to twelve at night and then be ready to go again early the next morning.

Like many people who work hard, Buzz also played hard and, unfortunately, this meant that he drank too much. Rarely did it interfere with his work, but it did interfere with his family life. After partying one day he and his lady partner drove down the road from Fort Ware, stopping on the way at a tree planters' camp. There they got into an argument with each other. When his girlfriend started to drive away, Buzz ran in front of the truck to stop her and ended up being run over and killed by his own truck.

His funeral service was held in Prince George and I was flabbergasted when his younger brother, Donny, asked if I would give the eulogy. I had done many different things while working for Fort Ware but this was a first for me, ever. The funeral home was crowded and the service unfolded as planned, including the playing of a song at full blast that had been a favourite of Buzz's. When I heard it, I wasn't sure how appropriate it was, but Donny said that it was Buzz's favourite piece and that it was the family's decision to play it: "Another One Bites the Dust"!

Some time later when I was driving from Fort Ware I met Donny, who was driving from Prince George. We had both stopped at Meselinka camp for coffee. I asked Donny where Buzz was buried. He startled me by answering, "Oh, he's in my truck." He indicated a box on the back seat.

"We cremated him and I'm taking the urn to Fort Ware and we'll bury him in the graveyard," Donny went on. "He's quite happy back there because he's next to a crate of beer!"

When I expressed my doubts about Antoine and Annie to Charlie Boya, he convinced me that they would be just fine on the trip and that he, Charlie, would vouch for them. He said there was no one better to take on a long hike than this couple, because they had spent their lives out in the bush, climbing mountains, hunting, hiking, and they also had well-trained pack dogs. I thought then that maybe I would learn some more about Sekani culture from them and how to really live in the bush (as long as it didn't involve making some kind of homebrew).

Another thing that concerned me was that Antoine was classified as legally blind. Years earlier, he had been working for BC Hydro or one of their contractors, clearing brush from the power line right-of-way. In spite of having safety equipment, his chainsaw had kicked back and resulted in an injury to his eye. I knew that he was able to hunt and trap, but whenever I met him in the store or on the street he had to peer at me from a few centimetres away through his Coke-bottle glasses so that he could identify me. This, however, was not a trip that was my responsibility and if I wanted to accompany the Sekani on the trail I had to trust Charlie's judgment. I also

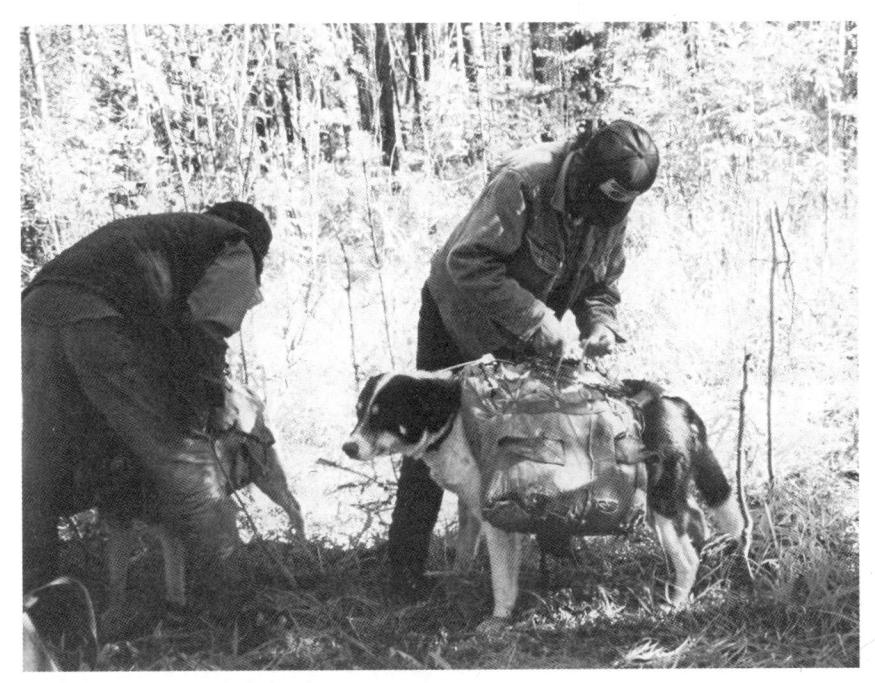

Charlie and Antoine saddle up the pack dogs.

remembered the positive things that I had heard around the village about Antoine's capabilities in the bush.

"And don't worry," Charlie said, "Annie is a good cook." Charlie knew he had me in a vulnerable spot. I did not like to go hungry. He said that Hazel would join us at Terminus Mountain and take over as cook.

In late summer, after attending an intertribal council meeting with Emil McCook in Ross River in the Yukon, I flew south to Watson Lake, where I had arranged to meet Charlie, Antoine and Annie. They had flown up to Watson Lake the previous day and had come out to the airport to meet me. Charlie's brother-in-law, Charlie Pete, a Tahltan who had lived in Lower Post for over thirty years, drove us from the airport down the Alaska Highway to Lower Post. There is some latent animosity between the Kaska and the Tahltan but I could never quite put my finger on the problem. Land claims, rivalry over work projects, protectionism, all seemed to bear on it.

According to the Yinka Dene Language Institute, the meaning of the name Kaska is an English adaptation of the Kaska name for McDame

Creek. The same word was borrowed for "Cassiar," the now-defunct town where tons of asbestos was mined and which was located in Kaska territory.

Because rivers were the main means of transportation in the past, houses were built in close proximity to this fluid highway. Lower Post, located just a hundred metres off the Alaska Highway, sprawls along the bank of the Liard River and no one is very far from the river. Old log buildings still exist, intermingled with newer houses that sport vinyl siding. A progressive plan was put in place so that a seniors' housing complex was built where entrances were shared to facilitate snow clearing. Later, a similar complex was built for single people and young couples that also had separate entrances. Most of the old residential school was torn down and what was left was converted into band offices. The band in Lower Post is still affiliated with the Liard Band in the Yukon and even though the bands agreed to separate, the federal government placed a moratorium on creating "new" bands. The Lower Post Band is thus officially "Liard River Band #3," but it is run quite autonomously. George Miller was instrumental in organizing the band council and later was a major player in the newly organized Kaska Tribal Council with Hammond Dick from Ross River serving as the Tribal Chief.

After we experienced an unexpected and delightful supper at the Petes' house, Charlie Pete arranged boat transportation for us to the starting point of the Davie Trail, a few kilometres up from the mouth of the Dease River. As we sat in the large kitchen, the conversation was quite confusing to follow because we had two Annies present: Annie Pete was married to Charlie Pete, and Annie Charlie was married to Antoine Charlie and then we had Charlie Boya. Unless you could catch someone's eye when you spoke to them, you could get either two different answers to your question or dead silence. It was easy to forget who had Charlie for a Christian name and who had Charlie for a surname and both Annies would answer to a question directed to one of them. I was glad that my name was Keith.

Annie Pete is Charlie Boya's sister. She had recently been Deputy Chief of Lower Post until her eyes were damaged in a car accident. Apparently all the Boyas had made a name for themselves in one way or another, and in witness to that, visitors who drive north on the Meziaden Highway pass the Boya Lake Provincial Park just north of Good Hope Lake, where there is a small Kaska village. Boya Lake was named for Louis Boya, Charlie Boya's father.

A local Kaska man, Malcolm Groat, brother of then Deputy Chief Debbie Groat of the Liard Band at Lower Post and a man who was an experienced river boat man, ferried us in his river boat from Lower Post across the Liard River to the head of the Davie Trail at Two Mile Cabin on the Dease River. We could feel strong eddies pulling the boat this way and that way as the two rivers joined forces. Malcolm expertly guided the boat through the whirls and eddies of first the Liard and then the Dease rivers. As the wind blew the hair in our faces, I could feel my excitement mounting and a certain amount of trepidation about starting out on a long hike.

These Boots Are Made for Walking

Through the trees, and nestled in a grassy clearing, were two log buildings surrounded by colourful fireweed. As we approached, I saw a large sign stating that this was the start of the Davie Trail and acknowledging the agencies that had sponsored the construction of the buildings and a few kilometres of trail-clearing. Several summer work projects had given a few Kaska youths some experience in trail-cutting. It had also given them the opportunity to camp and live in the bush and gain some knowledge they might not otherwise have acquired. We were to benefit from the few kilometres of trail they had cleared.

Steering his river boat slowly against the current, Malcolm brought it expertly up to the riverbank where there was a small gravel beach. We soon unloaded the supplies and hauled them up to the main cabin. As we waved goodbye to Malcolm, we surveyed the mountain of supplies that would need to be carried by the four of us, along with our four pack dogs. Charlie, Antoine and Annie did not seem to be at all perturbed by it all, so I relaxed too. We had brought two rifles and I had a satellite telephone with a solar charger, "just in case." Since I would be carrying one of the rifles and the satellite phone, I felt that I had enough insurance for the trip. We did not carry a GPS or even a compass so we were going to rely completely on what we could find of the trail and Charlie's guiding abilities.

We spent the evening sorting our supplies in the last of the evening sunlight and packing what we could into our packs. My pack weighed in at about 31 kg at the airport and we had weighed one of Antoine's dog packs at 20 kg. We carried only dried food for both ourselves and the dogs, and hoped to supplement this with grouse or perhaps a small deer. I tried not to think about what we would do if there were a shortage of game animals. There is a saying that animal tracks make pretty weak soup.

The evening seemed to stretch out, with the sun still high in the sky at nine o'clock. When we had finished our chores, we relaxed and sat by our campfire, staring at the flames and talking as we watched the Dease River flowing calmly by. The smoke from our campfire drifted out over the river and I thought of the river travellers who had been passing this way for many years. Since the cabins were built, people travelling by canoe had stopped here, probably to freshen up after weeks on the river and before arriving at a civilized community. One traveller from Germany had written his name and address on a log wall, citing his starting point and then his intended destination, the Liard Hot Springs. I was reminded of the many cabins with similar messages and comments that I had seen over the years. I wondered how many people these days added a felt pen to their list of necessary items as they prepared for a wilderness trip, because so many messages were written with the unmistakable heavy black ink.

Our pack dogs sat on beds of dry grass in the shade of the aspen trees, watching and listening to us, as if they knew that they had to rest. I wondered if they could sense the excitement when we had travelled with them in the planes. They watched quietly as we packed quantities of food and equipment into bags. These dogs were of no particular breed. Antoine's two dogs were big and strong and he used them for packing on a regular basis when he was at home in Fort Ware. The oldest, Boney, was a large black and white dog that almost looked as though he had some malamute in him. He always stayed close to Antoine and would push other dogs, or us, out of the way so that he could walk behind his master. The only time that Boney misbehaved was when he smelled wild game. Then he would start to get a bit agitated, then excited, and if a moose was quite close, Antoine said that Boney had been known to take off after it, sometimes coming back with his pack under his belly and sometimes without the pack at all. But he always came back "eventually," Antoine added with a smile.

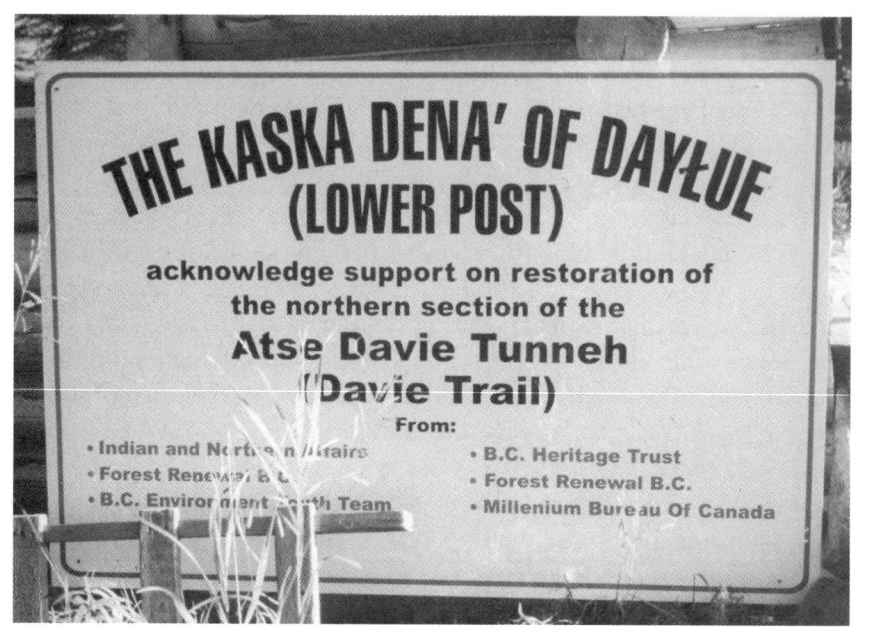

THE KASKA DENA' OF DAYŁUE (LOWER POST)
acknowledge support on restoration of the northern section of the
Atse Davie Tunneh (Davie Trail)
From:
- Indian and Northern Affairs
- Forest Renewal B.C.
- B.C. Environment Youth Team
- B.C. Heritage Trust
- Forest Renewal B.C.
- Millenium Bureau Of Canada

A sign posted by the Kasa Dena' marks the start of the Aatse Davie Trail.

Blackie, Antoine's second dog, was part wolf and jet black, as his name implied. He was identical to his mother, a pure black wolf, who had been raised at Ingenika after a litter of wolf pups had been found abandoned in a freshly logged area. She was intentionally mated with a local breed dog and Antoine had obtained Blackie as a pup from her litter. It did not seem to matter how big Blackie's pack was, or how heavy, he just did not seem to notice that it was there and was always willing to get up and go whenever Annie or Antoine moved.

Charlie had brought two of his dogs. Bruno, of German shepherd stock, was a very friendly, hard-working dog, that I knew well. Bruno often attached himself to me, and Charlie fastened him close to my tent at night, which made me sleep easier, especially in densely wooded country. Jimbo looked like someone's pet collie. A rather hairy dog with big floppy ears and a good nature, he was getting on in years, so Charlie gave him a smaller pack that was much lighter than the other dogs' loads. He had worked with Charlie on many trips, but perhaps he was more like me, past his prime.

Last but not least, and rather surprisingly, we had Annie's pet poodle, Tiny, along for the trip. Tiny was about as big as a rabbit, with long curly hair. She was just about the last thing I had expected to see on a long trek, but

Annie was not going to leave home without her. She called Tiny her bear dog and she stayed by Annie all the time—unless she decided to take off after the impossible dream, a squirrel, which she would chase after, yapping like a mad thing as she watched the squirrel jumping from tree to tree. She would go berserk when it stopped on a branch and scolded everyone. When the going got wet or when her little pooch tired, Annie would pack Tiny into her coat and carry her, her curly head poking out of the front of Annie's jacket. The funniest thing I saw was when Annie made a small, fitted dog pack for Tiny that would only hold a small tin of chewing tobacco. Her pet ran around with it, glancing over her back at this insult thrust upon her, as if Annie was trying to make her into a common pack dog!

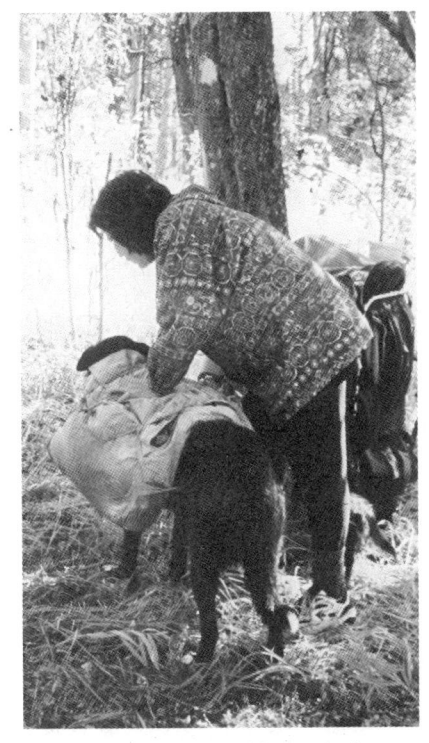

Annie Charlie loads up the pack dog Blackie.

When we finally turned in for the night, we were glad to see that there were some foam mattresses rolled up and hung from the cabin rafters. We laid them out on the plywood bunk beds in the cabins and enjoyed our last night in comparative comfort.

Watch Out for Bear!

I awoke early the next morning to the sound of Antoine cutting wood for the fire that we needed to cook our breakfast. The sun was already shining and a few fluffy white clouds drifted lazily across the blue sky. The sweet smell of wood smoke from the newly kindled fire assailed my nostrils, a smell that permeated all my belongings before many days had gone by, something that I was not really aware of until I was out of the camp environment at the end of the trip.

Antoine looked up at me through his thick glasses as I emerged from the cabin and smiled his shy smile. "Good morning, Keith," he said. I replied with a greeting and then watched as he returned to his task of splitting wood, which he did effortlessly. There was already more than enough wood split, but Antoine always left wood ready for the next travellers, who might be either freezing cold or exhausted when they arrived. After washing in the river, I returned to the cabin and found water already boiling in the kettle and ready for tea.

Annie had joined Antoine by the fire and she was stirring the breakfast of oatmeal "mush" in a blackened pan over the fire. Annie was quite a small woman, and proved to be very tough and bush-wise. She laughingly showed me her T-shirt, which had emblazoned across the front: "Canada, our home and NATIVE land." I had to laugh, and Charlie called out that I was about to see a lot more really traditional Native land.

Very few First Nations people that I knew openly expressed how much they resented being confined to Indian Reserves and forcibly made to attend residential schools, where they could not speak their native tongue or even converse with their siblings of the opposite sex. But as I became a familiar figure in the villages, and they realized that I was working for them and not for some far-off bureaucracy, they opened up their thoughts to me to such an extent that I felt a lot of sympathy about the injustices that had been done to them. Annie's T-shirt seemed like her way of making a statement about this. Farther down the trail, I was to see where Charlie and his sisters had been picked up unexpectedly from their home by the authorities, taken miles away to a residential school and separated from each other and their parents for years.

After a quick breakfast of the mush Annie had made, we packed our sleeping bags and then, as the last vestiges of our camp were dismantled, at Charlie's suggestion I set out on the well-defined trail. Charlie said they would soon catch up with me after tying the packs on the eager dogs, who were now standing wagging their tails furiously in anticipation of setting out on the trail. I was soon striding out on the start of the 460-kilometre Davie Trail. Glancing at my watch, I saw that it was only eight o'clock.

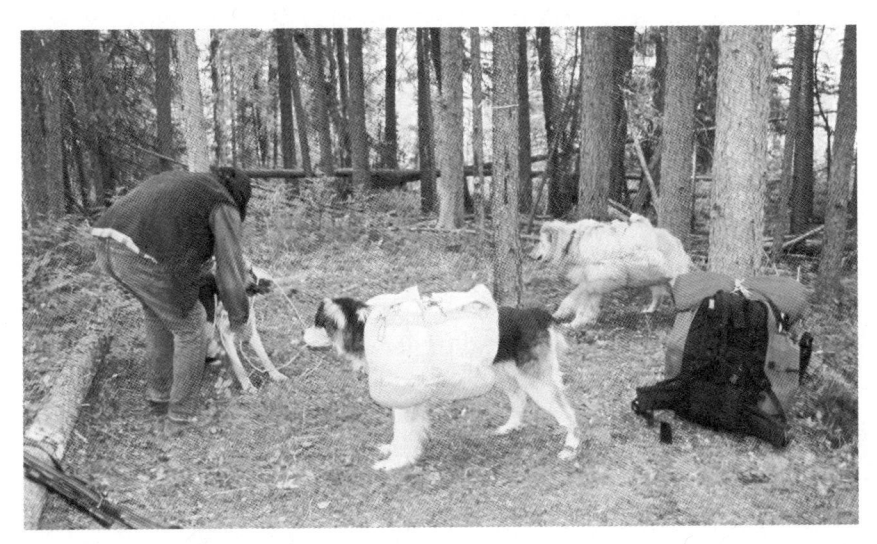

Three pack dogs, saddled up and ready to go.

92   Tse-loh-ne

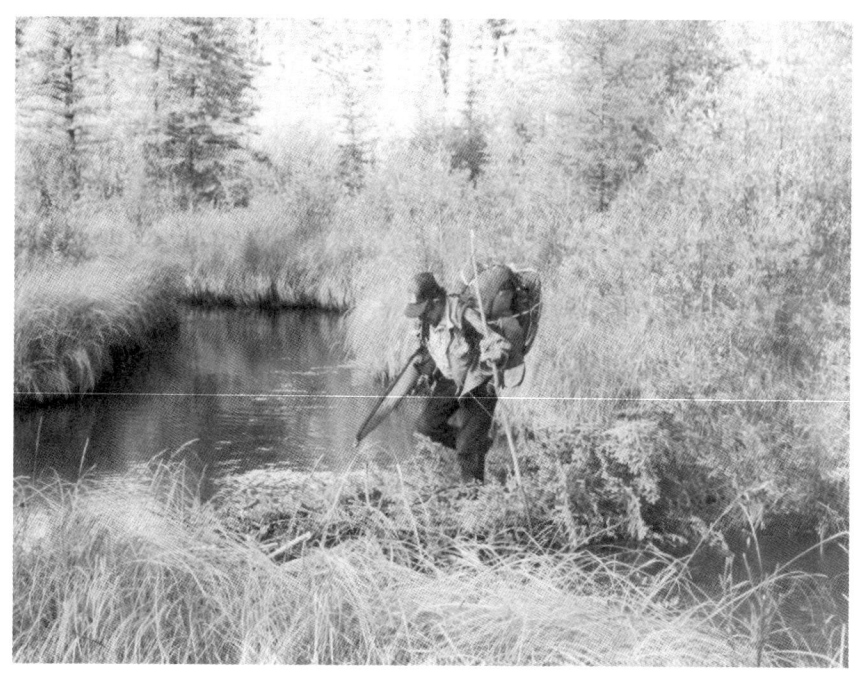

Antoine Charlie, who is legally blind, navigates a narrow bridge.

For the first few kilometres, the trail was marked with small orange discs with "Davie Trail" etched on them in white. They were nailed to trees every ninety metres or so. Eric Gunderson, under contract with the Kaska Tribal Council, had previously been down this part of the trail, putting up identification discs as he went along. He had turned off the Davie Trail after a few kilometres and headed west towards McDames, where he then had to wait for someone to come along and ferry him, his crew and their horses across the Liard River so that they could return to Watson Lake.

The ghost village of McDames, originally a gold mining claim and later a Hudson's Bay Company trading post, is located ten kilometres south of Good Hope Lake and a four-wheel drive along a rough trail leads to the Dease River. The trail that Eric had been on heads eastward to Birches Lake from McDames. A prospector, Harry McDame, thought to be a man of colour, had discovered gold on the small creek in 1874 and the post was named after him. A single large, windowless log building, a relic built by the Hudson's Bay Company, is all that is left of this once-important way station on the Dease River. I thought about the possibility that this was the site of the Hudson's Bay "Upper Post," being upriver from "Lower Post" since there seems to be no

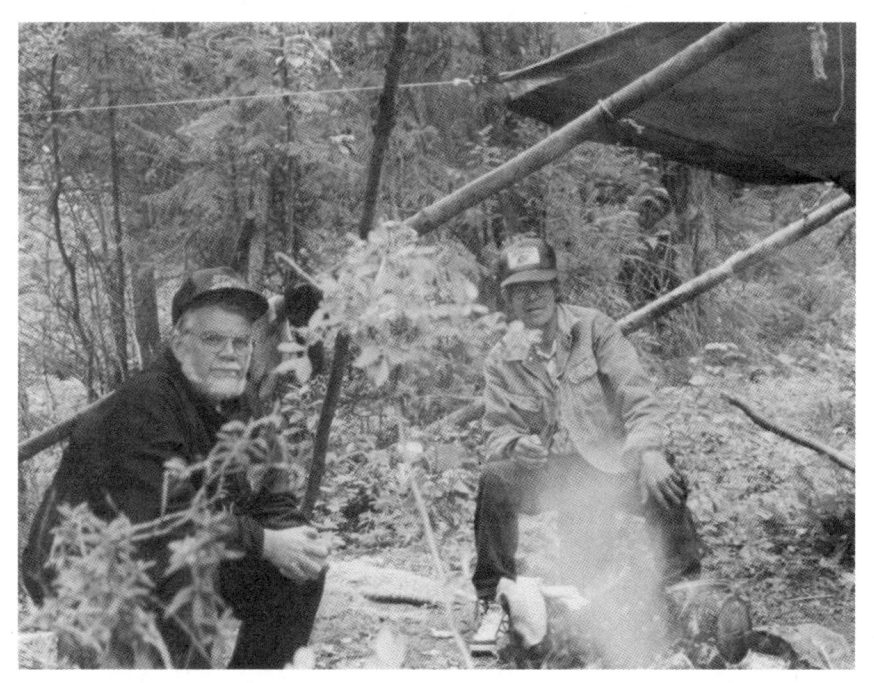

Keith and Antoine at camp.

site further down the Dease River that would answer. The lone building looks out over the river. On the opposite bank, there are the remains of a Native village, where wooden houses have collapsed under many winters of heavy snow and are now disappearing as the bush reclaims the land.

As though to symbolize the decay of McDames, there is a fenced graveyard set on a high bluff. There are a few fenced-in graves and one imposing stone monument. Its epitaph reads "In Memory of Webster Scott Simpson, Indian Agent, Died July 20 1927 on Dease River, B.C. 'Doing His Duty'," as if to remind the infrequent visitors to this site that it was once a thriving small community.

On this visit to McDames, I could see small trees growing inside the graveyard fences. Plans were being made to clear the land because the whole area has a historical significance and possible tourist value. While exploring the store site with some Fort Ware Band members a few years ago, we came across a huge river barge that was partly hidden, lying rotting in the bushes. It was built in the style of the local river boats, but bigger than the old York boats that the Hudson's Bay Company used. We could only imagine the freight capacity of the boat, and were left wondering who or what had powered it.

As I continued down the Davie Trail, the well-worn pathway was mostly free of fallen logs and other brush and reminded me of a park trail. The path wandered through rolling hills where stands of small spruce trees were interspersed with small deciduous trees and berry bushes. My pack was heavy but it did not impede my progress and I briefly thought of Samuel Black's men travelling to the Turnagain River carrying packs that weighed 54 kg (120 lbs).

The heavy pack I carried was light compared to what the Sekani in the nineteenth century packed when they hired out as packers, carrying furs or supplies. By comparison I was carrying pocket change. According to the BC Archives, their packs were unbelievably heavy:

> The standard pack weight for men was 45 kg. On top of this the packer would have his own food and supplies for the trip. The standard pack for women was "only" 36 kg. Many times on top of their large packs, they would have blankets, food and a baby. Packers would receive five cents per 0.45 kg for the supplies they carried. In the 1860s, for the trip from Hazelton to Fort Babine, a distance of almost 160 km both ways, the packer was paid only $4.00 or $5.00.

I naively thought that if the trail was going to be as easy all the way as the first few kilometres were, we could reach the Kechika River in a week. Once the countryside had enveloped us, though, I noticed that the trail disc markers were farther apart, there was more vegetation growing on the trail and the log bridges gave way to swampy crossings.

My pack began to dig into my shoulders as I walked along the trail in the dappled sunlight but I felt a spring in my stride. I fully expected the first few days to be physically tough, because as usual, and against all the advice I received, I had done nothing to prepare my body for what it was expected to do—I had been too busy with office work.

The bush gave off a slowly decaying aroma of late summer or early fall, and the trees were just beginning to change their bright green mantle for more sombre yellows and browns. I eased off my pack and swung my arms around and felt how good it was to be out on a trail again. I shouldered my pack again, picked up my rifle, and set off down the trail, enjoying the fresh morning air, walking at my own pace. I noticed fresh moose tracks along the trail, some black bear spoor, and scat signs from both wolf and fox. Spruce grouse or ptarmigan had walked along the trail leaving their worm-like feces to tantalize any hungry predator that came along.

As I started to climb a long hill, I heard a noise some way behind me, and I resolved to get up the hill before the others caught up to me. As I reached the top, I saw that the trail ahead branched both right and left. Unsure which way to go, and hearing some panting on the trail behind me, I turned to ask Charlie for directions. Instead of Charlie, I stood facing a large black bear, standing less than two metres away.

That's Life on the Trail!

The bear stopped when I stopped and just looked at me when I turned around, weaving his head from side to side and snapping his teeth together, a dangerous sign. Without really thinking about it, I dropped my pack to the ground and got my rifle out of the scabbard, all in the blink of an eye, and there we stood, looking at each other. I yelled at the bear to go away, but he continued his unnerving teeth mashing—as if he couldn't wait to sink them into me. I wondered whether I should shoot him in the head or the chest if he took a run at me, but, at the same time, I was hoping that the others would arrive and save the day. I was sweating profusely with the exertion of walking up the hill and now with nervous apprehension, and it crossed my mind that sour smells attract bears to a likely food source—and I didn't want to be on his menu.

The bear was the first to break the impasse. Making my heart pound even more, with a snort, he ran into some cranberry bushes just to my right. There he peered at me through the bush. Now he was about four metres away—a small improvement—but my legs still felt weak. I could hardly believe that I was face to face with a bear this early on in the trip. If this was just the first day, what would the rest be like? I kept my rifle pointing at him, not wanting to shoot, but if it came to a life or death decision, I knew which side I wanted to be on.

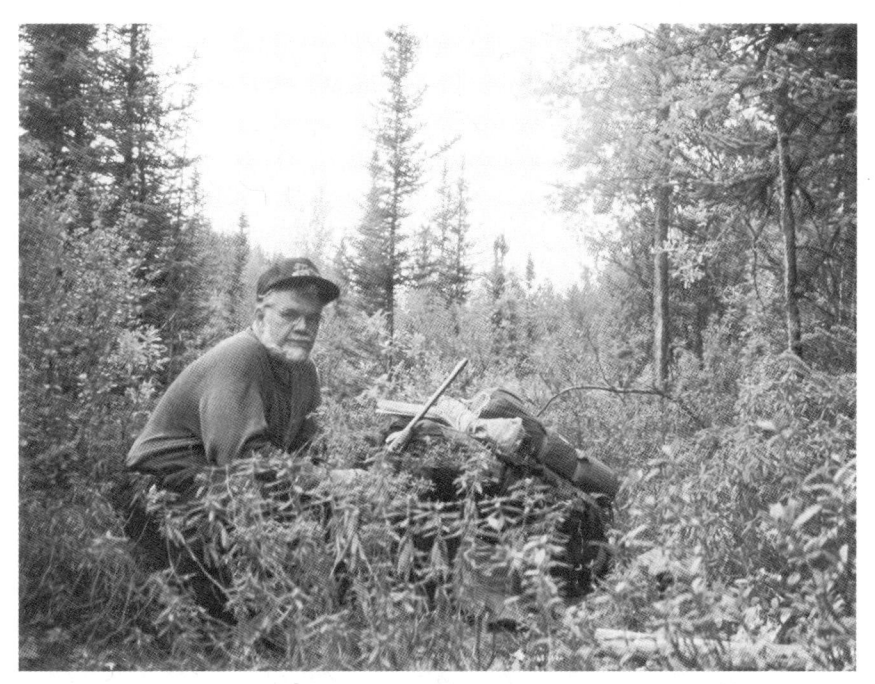

Keith, who has just been confronted by a black bear, takes a moment to recover.

I could see the bear's beady black eyes looking at me through the bush, but now he was very quiet and still. Was this good or bad? The books say that if you are confronted by a bear do not look him in the eye. Ha! When you are confronted with a bear in real life you are not going to look up at the clouds. You are going to watch him carefully, and if he is as short-sighted as the same books say, he won't know whether you are looking him in the eye or at his rear end. As it was, and to my great relief, the bear uttered a contemptuous snort, turned, and pounded off through the small spruce trees. I could hear him crashing through the underbrush for several seconds afterwards.

I kept my eyes turned in the direction where the noise was coming from, but relaxed my grip on the rifle. As I was staring into the bush, another noise behind me made me swing around. To my relief, I saw Charlie appear with Antoine and Annie. I tried to sound calm and asked him which trail we should take. He looked at my gun questioningly, so I told him about the bear. Annie said that a bear would sometimes follow someone down a trail because they were just plain curious, but I was not convinced that my encounter had been only with a curious bear. Charlie had seen fresh bear scat on the trail and had assumed that the bear was most probably ahead of me and that I had scared him off the trail. When we were ready again, I shouldered my pack, picked up my gun and followed Charlie along the trail, happy to be with some human company again.

Charlie set a fast pace and we all dutifully followed him. The dogs followed us with tongues hanging out and tails held high. Jimbo, at thirteen years old, was quite slow and soon we lost sight of him. Charlie said that he would catch up to us eventually.

After a break for some lunch, Charlie told me to go ahead again since the trail was well marked. They would soon catch up with me, but he wanted to wait for Jimbo and let the other dogs have a few more minutes' rest. "And watch out for bears!" he said with a laugh.

The map showed numerous creeks along the way so we hadn't packed any drinking water. Later in the day, we had to assume that the creeks—Liard Tom Creek, Kloye Creek and Trepanier Creek—had all dried up in the hot, dry weather, and we were soon wracked with thirst. Swamp water was visible in some areas that we passed, but we didn't want to risk drinking anything stagnant. The dogs, on the other hand, were not fussy and lapped up anything that looked wet.

I was walking ahead again, and came to a small clearing in the middle of a stand of jackpine that had obviously been used as a campsite some time ago. There were a few blackened rocks in the centre of the clearing and some half-burned logs scattered around. Through the trees, I could see a large body of water. I checked my map and saw that it must be Black Angus Creek, which had been flooded by a beaver dam. We had hiked over seventeen kilometres, so I knew we would be stopping here at least for a rest. I changed from my wet socks, glad to see that so far there were no blisters. I cut some wood and made a fire, but Antoine had the kettle with him so I couldn't make any tea. Instead, I just rested and fed the fire until my three friends arrived a short time later with three of the dogs. The dogs sat down and patiently watched us, glad to have a rest from carrying their packs. We noticed that Jimbo had not caught up and later, as we sat and drank tea, Charlie said that he was going to go back and look for him.

Antoine said that even though it was early, about mid-afternoon, we should make camp while we were close to water, and it was with some relief that I was soon lying in my tent on my sleeping bag and resting my aching legs. Antoine took the kettle and another pot down to the creek for more water. Annie said that the problem with stopping early was that the evenings were then so long. She felt that it would be better to start later in the mornings.

Charlie came back to camp several hours later with Jimbo, having walked almost halfway back along the trail calling his name.

To dampen our spirits, a steady drizzle began to fall and before long, everything that wasn't under the tarpaulin we had rigged up was soaked. It was still light, so Charlie and Antoine decided to go for a walk down the trail. Annie mended some dog packs, then tidied up the camp before settling down to read a book. I kept the fire going and a pot of water boiling for tea.

During the night, the dogs all started to bark and I heard

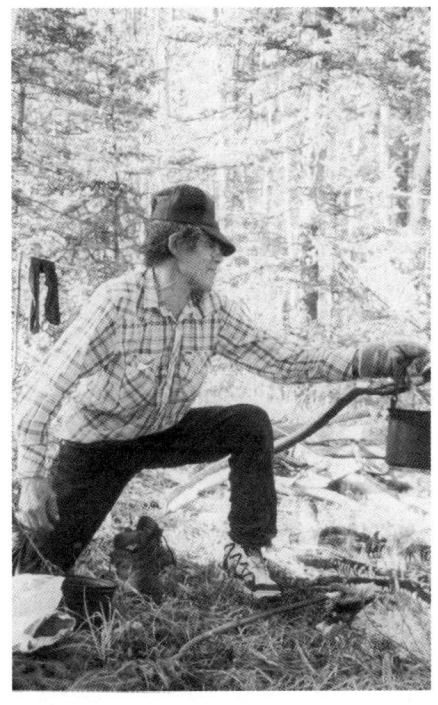

Antoine boils the kettle for tea.

Antoine shout at them to shut up. I thought maybe some wolves or a bear had ventured close by, but having the dogs tied up around the camp gave me a feeling of security and I soon fell asleep again.

As usual, I awoke to the sounds of Antoine cutting wood for the fire. As I peered out of my tent, I could see that the fire was already blazing and the black tea kettle was beginning to sing, a very pleasant sound first thing in the morning. The day was cloudy but the rain had stopped and water hung on every leaf sparkling in the morning light. After a breakfast of oatmeal and a cup of tea, we packed up and set out on the trail again. The wet leaves soon lost their sparkling attraction for me as the rainwater ran off them as we passed and quickly soaked into my clothes.

After walking along low, wet, spongy terrain, we started to climb to slightly higher ground where the trail was dry and had a dry layer of spruce needles covering it. We had not had much of a view because the trees were thick and there was no real high ground, just undulating hillocks. As we came to a low ridge, we found an old, abandoned dog sleigh. It was long and narrow, with its handlebars still intact but one runner was missing. It was in the final stages of decay and lay beside what looked like an old camp or small cabin, with a few rotting logs, the remains of a wall. It was hard to picture what kind of structure the fallen logs represented.

This was the section of the trail that Charlie's father, Louis Boya, had used many years ago when he travelled between his trapline at Islands Lake and his home in Lower Post. Charlie wondered aloud if this had been his father's sleigh. He said that in the springtime his father would leave the trapping cabin with the winter's furs and, using his sled dogs, would set out for Lower Post to trade the furs. When he ran out of snow, the sled would be cached and he would continue with his dogs now packing his supplies on their backs, just as our dogs were packing some of our supplies for us now.

We descended into thick willows that could give you a stinging slap in the face if you followed too close to the person in front of you. Consequently, we travelled with our heads down to escape being whipped. After several hours of walking on the twisting and turning trail, alternating between high, dry hills, and low-lying swamp, we found that the trail just disappeared. We had travelled about seven kilometres, according to my pedometer. Charlie was annoyed with himself for not looking for tree blazes as he walked along.

Charlie normally had an uncanny sense of direction when out in the bush, but put him in the city and he would easily get lost. He once got on a bus in Prince George to go several blocks, though he didn't know that his destination was really that close. When he couldn't recognize anything, he just kept riding the bus and ended up touring the city. When the bus driver told him that he would have to get off, Charlie was surprised to find himself back at his starting point. As we looked around for signs of the trail, I wanted to remind him that he wasn't on a bus in Prince George now, but the mood of the moment prevented me from saying anything.

We had slowed down considerably as we gazed around and when we saw a small mossy area, Charlie heaved off his pack and told us what I wanted to hear. We would make camp. The dogs sank down on the moss and lay there panting and licking their paws. We all helped unload the dogs and tied them up to individual trees, making sure that they wouldn't get tangled up in the bushes. We emptied the dog packs and then hung them up to dry.

The packs, which sat on either side of the dogs' backs, were made of heavy canvas and moosehide and were almost as long as the dog's body. They were tied on with light rope, one rope around the dog's neck, another under its tail, and then the packs were tied around the dog's middle. This was similar to the way packs were placed and tied on horses with a diamond hitch. This prevents the pack from sliding forward as the dog goes down a steep hill or riverbank, and the same applies when the dog goes up a hill or jumps over a fallen tree. Most of the time it worked, but in thick bush the packs sometimes slid around to the dog's belly, making it almost impossible for the dog to walk.

After Charlie had put up a tarp and unpacked his sleeping blanket, he said that he would go ahead and make sure he knew where the trail was and find out if we had gone wrong. He admitted that being away from the mountains was disconcerting because he had no real landmarks to give him a sense of direction, and since the trail traversed this plain at the end of the Rocky Mountains, there was nothing but trees around us. Since Charlie had only travelled this part of the trail when he was a youngster, it did not look very familiar to him. In the intervening years, rivers and creeks had changed their course and trees had grown larger or died, and the trail had changed accordingly. This was no different from when I went back to one of the cities I had lived in years ago, and finding the roads and buildings all changed, got lost in what had once been very familiar surroundings.

I had brought along what I thought was a reasonably good map and we had been given a copy of a map of the northern area by the Kaska Tribal Council. I also tried to estimate the distance that we were travelling with my pedometer, and dutifully marked the map with our location every night.

While Antoine and I cut some firewood, Annie made a nicely browned fry-pan bannock. She added more rice to a pack of dehydrated chicken soup and cooked it up. Along with some beef jerky I had brought along, we were soon enjoying a good meal.

Charlie came back to camp without finding where the trail might have branched off, and said that he should go back and search for Jimbo again. Later, when he returned, he said that in spite of walking a long way back, there was no sign of his dog, and that Jimbo had possibly lain down in some bushes off the trail, or had turned around and gone back to the cabin on the Dease River. As evening came on, we heard wolves howling in the distance and Annie voiced the opinion that the wolves in the area might get him. Charlie felt that there was nothing else that he could do that night. Jimbo was carrying some of our rice, dry dog food, some jam and bits and pieces that Charlie had crammed into the pack, things we could manage without if Jimbo didn't show up, but I could tell he was concerned about his dog.

I have heard people talk about wolves sometimes mating with a loose dog but a friend of mine in Fort St. James had a bad experience that seemed to disprove that. He was travelling sixty kilometres to his trapline cabin by snowmobile and had let his sled dogs run behind him along the trail. The snowmobile soon outdistanced the dogs but their owner didn't worry because the dogs knew the trail well and would follow on. By next morning the dogs had not arrived at the cabin, so he went to look for them on his snowmobile. He came to a section of his trail that was covered with wolf tracks and, as he looked around, he found a piece of harness, then a dog collar and looking further, he saw dog hair and some gnawed sections of one of his dog's legs. A northern British Columbia wolf is easily as big as a Newfoundland dog, but much sleeker and stronger. On the other hand, Antoine had Blackie, who had wolf in his bloodlines but from a semi-domesticated animal. We were all concerned for Jimbo because he was such a cute dog and hearing the wolves made us feel very uneasy. A steady rain began to fall that seemed to match our dampened spirits.

Charlie left early the next morning to scout for the trail. He was sure that there must be signs of it somewhere close by. In what seemed like a very short time, he came back and said he had found the trail, which was well hidden amongst some aspen trees in a place where beavers had flooded a large area. Using his axe, Charlie had cut a way around the newly created

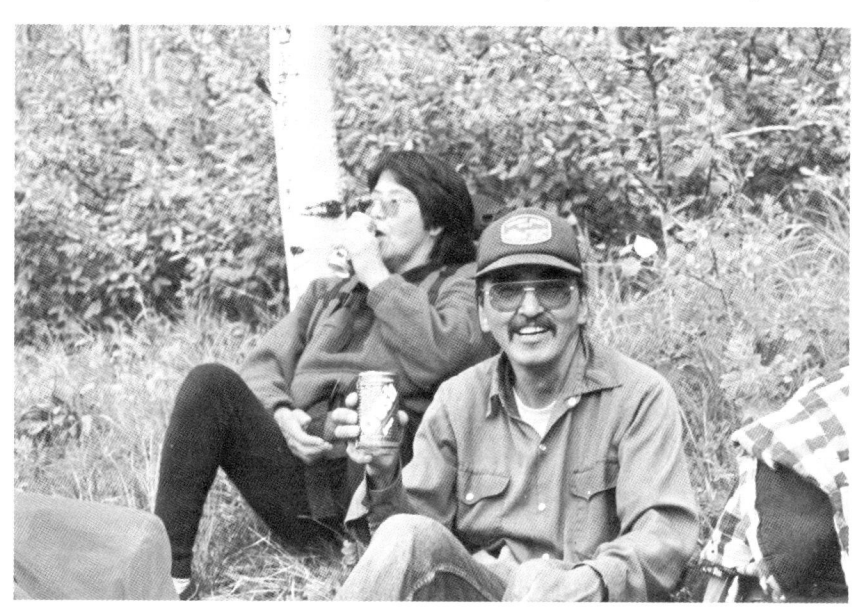

Hazel and Charlie lighten their packs.

swamp so we could get the dogs through without soaking their packs and without us having to wade.

We left camp at nine-thirty in the morning as the clouds began to roll away. Still no sign of Jimbo. (A couple of weeks after we had returned home, Charlie had a call from Malcolm Groat to say that Jimbo had returned to the cabin on the Dease River and someone had taken him to Lower Post, where he was now living.) It was not raining, but everywhere was wet and the bushes showered us as we walked by. The trail alternated between soggy, muddy swamp in the low, flat areas and then, as we climbed higher, it became drier, covered with spruce needles that made it soft and very pleasant to walk on.

We descended to a small, fast-flowing stream that we thought should be Kaska Creek. Too wide and deep to jump across, Charlie and Antoine soon found two pine trees close to the water's edge and expertly felled them across the creek, using the branches to make something resembling a deck. Before long, we were able to cross over easily without having to unload the dogs.

The country we were now travelling through consisted of a series of hills and gullies which gave our leg muscles a good workout as we struggled up the hills to the dry trails and then came down again to the swampy, bushy, foot-sucking muskeg. As we climbed higher again, the trail became drier, but there were always deadfalls to clamber over.

This up and down, wet and dry pattern seemed to fill our days and as we plodded on, I tried to visualize the early travellers coming down the trail. What were they looking forward to? Did they worry about having enough food? Did they travel in wet moccasins every day? Were they patient with the elderly and the very young? Did they complain to each other about the wet, the flies? Did they ever think about what was going on in the world "out there"? Were they even aware of or bothered about other parts of the country or were they absorbed in their own lives? Did they travel along in silence, only remarking on animal signs and such?

The weather improved considerably and before long we were walking under a blue sky. In spite of the earlier rain and the swamps that we had passed through, there were very few mosquitoes to bother us, a fact that relieved me. When you are pushing through the bush and sweating profusely, mosquitoes will normally come long distances to feed on any exposed skin. I had read that a female mosquito will travel for twenty kilometres in search of blood, but there were very few around now, not even in the evening, when hordes of them usually appeared. We were sometimes pestered by small blackflies, but they didn't bite. They would land on any exposed skin, even if insect repellent had been applied, and just sit there.

Wherever there were natural meadows, we found signs of old camps, with tree blazes that looked to be about fifty years old. People like the packer Skook Davidson, whose lodge site we would come to farther down the trail, would have used these areas to stop and let his horses rest and eat.

Although the rain had abated by late afternoon, we could see thunderheads piling up on the horizon, and peals of thunder reverberated in the distant mountains, making the dogs' ears twitch and swivel like small radar scanners, as they tried to locate the source.

Nearly all the wild flowers we saw had gone to seed, although a scattering of dark blue lupines contrasted sharply with surrounding wild shasta daisies that were just beginning to look a bit dried out. Under the trees, where it was dry and devoid of undergrowth, grey lichens grew and old man's beard hung from the trees—an enticing food for woodland caribou.

The rolling hills and deep clefts where a river or creek had cut through thousands of years ago made it easy to imagine a covering of ice that slowly crept southwards, carving and shaping land as it moved down towards the Rocky Mountains, leaving this vast alluvial plain. Geologists say that there were some areas called Beringia that were not covered by ice because the climate was too dry and instead was home to the mammoth, giant bear and the scimitar cat, who fed on the grasses and plants that grew on this hard, cold land. The remains of these beasts have been found and are now on display in Whitehorse. It is said that the Native peoples came over to Beringia from Siberia when the Bering Sea had dried up and they survived by hunting these large animals. It is interesting to note that the language of the First Nations people is Athapascan, and there are similarities in the various dialects all the way from the Gwich'in in the far north to some of the First Nations people of Mexico. A large building in Whitehorse is now the display centre for Beringia information and fossils.

It is difficult to imagine what the land would have looked like then. Certainly if there were any trees, they would have been small stunted specimens. As we walked through this still-rugged country, we found that some of our campsites were quite idyllic, a haven for us after slogging through swamps or forcing our way through tangled willows that surrounded an old beaver dam. We came upon one such campsite after travelling only twelve kilometres through some tough countryside. We stepped out of heavy overgrowth onto a narrow, clear trail in a picturesque setting where a small lake

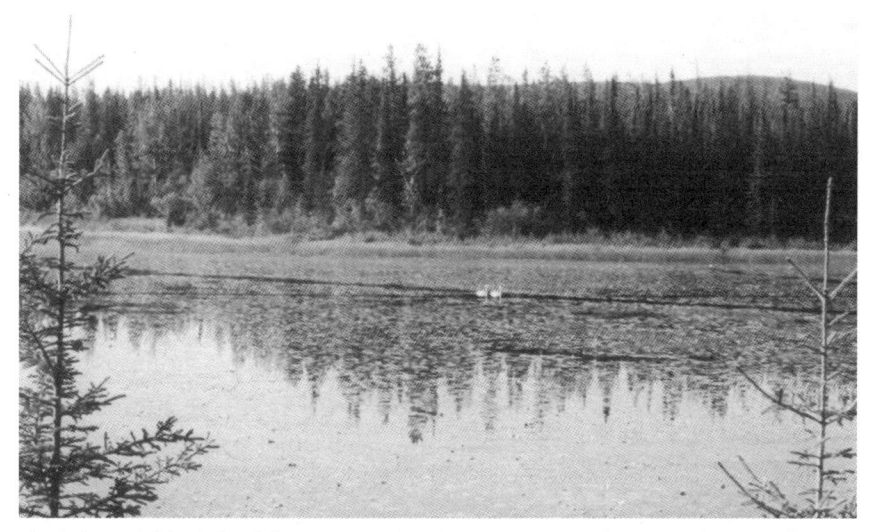

The hikers dubbed this lake "Swan Lake" because it was the only place on the trip where they encountered swans.

was surrounded by tall bulrushes and a clearing covered with wild hay. Two swans could be seen gracefully swimming across the mirrored surface of the lake, their wake sending small ripples dancing towards the shore. A large new beaver house had been built on one side of the lake and beaver trails led down from well-gnawed stumps of deciduous trees through the reeds and grasses to the water's edge. To complete the picture, two loons were seen swimming through the calm waters, which meant that the lake had fish in it. Unfortunately we hadn't brought anything to fish with. We decided to call this small lake "Swan Lake" because it was the only time that we saw swans. Antoine found three recently used moose beds, and said they were probably from a cow moose with twin calves. Although we couldn't see a creek, we estimated that we were near Mustela Creek. When we had set up camp and eaten a prepackaged dehydrated dinner (by this time I could have eaten the back end of one of Skook's pack horses!), Charlie went to scout ahead and found that we would have to cross a couple of beaver dams and then find a way over Mustela Creek.

The thunderheads had passed over us but then an ominous dark cloud positioned itself overhead. As if to make sure we did not get too comfortable, it started raining heavily. The sky to the west was brighter and since the wind was coming from that direction we hoped the storm would soon blow over and leave us in peace at our "Swan Lake."

By morning the sky was clear again but the ground was sodden. It was the same every day: we started out with dry boots and socks and then, after a few minutes of walking, would feel water permeate our socks and squish between our toes. At least the water felt warm. My right lower leg, probably the calf muscle, was painful and made me limp. I had to smile as I walked up a hill, turning my foot slightly inwards to ease the pain, and bent almost double with my heavy pack—I must have looked like Quasimodo out for a stroll!

For the most part, there were old tree blazes to follow, but now and again as if to throw us off, we saw side trails that had also been blazed, and it took an observant eye to recognize the main trail. By lunchtime, we came to the end of the frequently blazed trees, and all afternoon we followed a very poorly defined trail. The old-timers would have stayed on the clearer ground even if it was swampy, because any trail that goes through forest needs continual upkeep and clearing because of fallen trees.

It was difficult to see some of the small blazes from fifty metres away, but I was surprised and thankful when Annie's sharp eyes kept calling out to us that she could see another one. We came to an area of willow and alder and then some old-growth pine trees. In the middle of these trees, jammed into the fork of a tree about two metres from the ground, I saw an old moose antler, most likely propped there by someone travelling the trail. Immediately after this we came to a small esker where the trees and bushes had been cleared along its spine, leaving enough room for a bus, and certainly more than enough room for hikers or horses. We followed this for about one and a half kilometres until it suddenly ended and we were back on the trail again. We were to see a similar sight on the southern portion of the trail that had supposedly been made by trail-cutters working for Charles Bedaux.

After walking about twenty-five kilometres that day, Charlie said that we would make camp when we came across some water. That seemed to guarantee that we wouldn't find any, and at six-thirty when my stomach was thinking that my throat had been cut, we came to a big slough at the side of the trail. Charlie threw down his pack and at last said that we would camp at this spot.

When the camp was set up, Annie said that her feet were sore and she felt cold, so she put out her sleeping blanket and went to sleep. I cooked and ate something called a "Backpackers Omelet," which was supposed to feed four according to the label, but unless it was meant for backpacking turtles, it was only enough for one. I did offer some to Antoine, but after looking at it and then asking what it was, he declined and made some kind of soup of his own.

Restless Charlie, in his inimitable style, walked down the trail to see what was around the bend, and came back shortly with a grouse he had shot out of a tree with a slingshot. After literally peeling the bird, Charlie threw the wings, skin, and feathers to one of the dogs, who promptly devoured everything. He boiled up the breast meat and shared it with Antoine after offering me some, but it was my turn to decline. They saved a small portion for Annie, who ate it with some tea when she woke up, saying she felt much better.

After six days on the trail, we began to think that the map we were using was not very accurate, since it did not show very many creeks, and yet we had passed by a few of them—most were dry, but they were definitely creeks. Willows and small trees grew along the creek beds, obviously relishing the small amount of water that they could get and yet only a few metres away, the ground was quite dry, with virtually no plant growth. With all the swamps we had been through and the rain we had experienced, it was surprising that the creeks were dry. Beaver had been very busy throughout the whole trail area and they may have dammed up the creeks. With the decline in trapping, the land was reverting to the pre-trapping conditions of several hundred years ago when these animals were overly abundant in the north.

Several times, when we passed a small creek, Charlie had asked me what the map said the name of it was, and I would answer that it should be Calf Creek. When we came to make camp by another creek, he asked again what the map showed this time. I studied the map with him and we looked around at the topography and then we both burst out laughing. It looked like we were at Calf Creek. This was now the second time that we said we were camping at Calf Creek. Whether it was or not was immaterial, since we could tell by the sun that we were heading in the right direction, and when we came to some high ground, we could see that we were getting closer to the mountains. This made Charlie feel more at ease.

Before maps were drawn by the early white explorers, the Native peoples of North America found their way around their territory by memory and word of mouth, and the information was passed down from generation to generation. Like Charlie Boya, the people who lived close to mountains had very obvious reference points, but the Inuit in the Northwest Territories found their way across countless miles of frozen ocean, sometimes using the wind direction or the snow dunes to keep them on course. An old man told

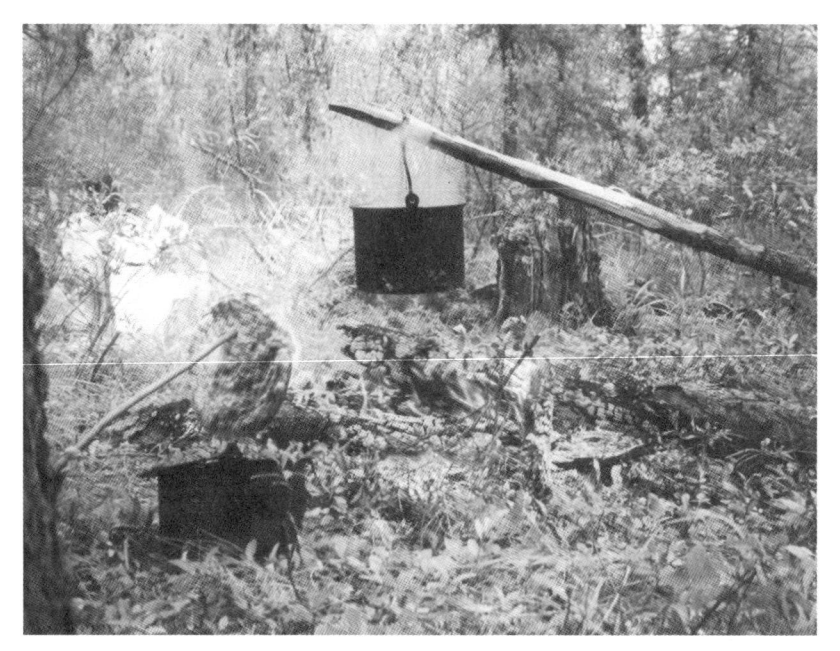

Tea and bannock. Now that's a feast!

me that during blizzards or white-outs he was conscious of direction from the direction the wind hit his nose, but when I tried that all I got was a frozen nose. In the city, I now find that I use various landmarks to give me reference points and I rarely look at the street signs. After living in the city for twenty years, I still can't give anyone directions using street names.

Charlie and I were walking ahead of Antoine and Annie when we saw a side trail. Charlie pointed to some traps hanging in a tree about two metres above the ground. The rusty traps looked as though they had not been used for years and were hanging on nails as though waiting for their owner to come and pick them up. Someone had evidently trapped here a long time ago and we wandered along the mossy trail discussing the probable owner. Charlie suggested some of the trappers he thought might have trapped here. It brought home to me the fact that someone had been out here in the middle of winter, braving the cold and the deep snow so that he could make a living, and travelling miles on snowshoes and camping in frigid temperatures. We were making our trip by choice, not necessity, and we didn't have family and children to worry about. Though we were sometimes wet, we were not contending with the cold. Another example of "the good old days!"

Just as we saw that the trapping trail was getting very narrow, we heard a faint shout from Annie. This brought me back to the present and alerted us as to how far we had wandered off the main trail, so we turned around and went back, rejoining the others.

A kilometre further on Antoine and Annie made camp after crossing a long beaver dam with their dogs, picking their way carefully over the logs, sticks and slippery mud. I followed Charlie across the beaver dam and got within two metres of the shore when I stepped into a hole and disappeared, with my pack on top of me.

Too Little, Too Much Water

My water bottle slipped away and I grabbed it as I saw it sliding past me down the muddy side of the dam. Meanwhile Charlie had reached the other side and walked off into the trees without noticing my disappearance. My leg seemed to be stuck fast between two logs. I struggled to get my arms out of the pack straps, feeling like a trussed-up chicken ready for the oven. With my heavy pack sitting on top of me, it was almost impossible to move. I tried moving my leg, and could have got out much more easily if I could have bent it the other way, but I didn't want to pull a muscle or worse, break my leg, so I rested a moment and thought about what to do.

My mind flitted from limb to limb, assessing the possibilities for movement. I thought that as surely as I had got into this hole, then just as surely, I could get out. I managed to get my arms onto some very wet logs and strained upwards. My leg was able to move slightly and I found an equally wet log that I could get my free knee on, then, an inch at a time, I manoeuvred myself until I could get one arm out of the pack strap, and then still inching my way up, I struggled to the top of the dam.

I looked at the virtual cage that had tried to hold me prisoner. It didn't look that bad. It was just an accident of nature that the beaver had placed his logs rather haphazardly, thereby reversing the roles of victim and trapper and managing to trap a human. When I thought of the helpless feeling that I was experiencing a moment before, I sympathized with any animal that was trapped. At least I didn't have an iron bar across my leg.

I finally reached the camp and related my experience to the group and we all had a good laugh. If I hadn't shown up, I know they would have come back for me, but they had just assumed that I had stopped for a bathroom break or to take a photograph. Since it all turned out well, there was nothing to do but laugh about it.

As I settled down on a bank of moss with my water bottle and prepared to take a long drink, nature again reminded me to be careful. I unscrewed the top of the bottle and as I raised it to my lips, I spied something wiggle to the top of the bottle. Peering in, I stared at what looked to me like a mosquito larva. I wondered how many I had swallowed during the day, but feeling very thirsty, I shook it out of the bottle and took a long draught. The water tasted okay and wasn't at all chewy.

During the day, Charlie had shot three more "chickens" with his slingshot and Annie fried them up for us, with a good helping of rice. The dogs shared what we didn't eat but Antoine said that his big dogs were getting hungry. The dry dog food was almost gone and he thought that they should try to get a beaver for meat for the dogs. Charlie took his rifle and walked down the trail to see if he could see anything, but Annie thought that it was too late in the day for a successful hunt.

Charlie returned about two hours later, having walked a long way without seeing any game although some game had seen him. On his return along the trail, Charlie saw signs that first a black bear had been following him and then later on he saw fresh grizzly bear scat on the trail. He was glad that he had his rifle with him, but saw nothing edible. Perhaps the bears had felt the same way.

Maybe because we were close to water and it was dusk, or because we were probably "ripe" after several wet, sweaty days on the trail, the blackflies became really bothersome, and for the first time, Annie hung a mosquito net from a tree so that she could read in peace. Charlie and Antoine went to cut more firewood, but when I went to help, I was told to go and rest. Sometimes I really felt like an old white man!

Before we had left Lower Post, Malcolm Groat, who seemed to be the only person who had any knowledge of the trail, had told us that there was a stretch of nearly sixteen kilometres without drinking water before we reached the Red River. Anticipating that we were within striking distance

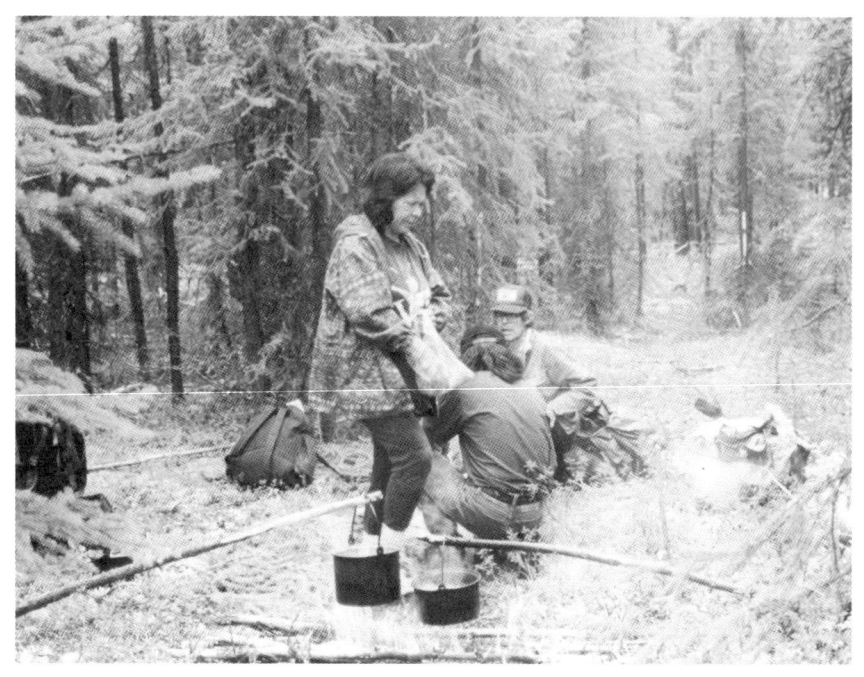

Annie Charlie was a great cook. Here she prepares lunch on the trail.

of the Red River, we filled up our water bottles before we left camp the next morning.

I was feeling unwell when we set out and started thinking about the water I had been drinking. Perhaps it was beaver fever, because it had been impossible to get any water that the beaver had not shared in some way. I had been quite diligent with my own sanitation, and I knew that Annie always took great care to wash her hands with soap and water before she cooked anything. She also used a Wash'n'Dry towelette to clean her hands again during food preparation. When you are on a backpacking trip, about the last thing you want is a bout of diarrhea. TP is not available in large quantities since it's bulky, and using moss is, uh, different—close attention to removing small sticks from the moss is very desirable!

The sun came out and it seemed to intensify the smell of the pine trees. This was very pleasant after the sour smell of the swamps, and made the rest of our morning trek very enjoyable. Before long, the hot sun was beating down upon us, and we were very thankful for the water that we carried and used sparingly. The dogs managed to find a few swampy puddles where they lapped up water greedily. We had run out of dog food by this time, but they kept on going, as strong as ever. Antoine promised them a good meal that night.

My stomach soon settled down, probably because any excess fluid was quickly sweated out, and after a rest stop, I walked on ahead while Charlie, Antoine and Annie were putting the packs back on the panting dogs. I kept my rifle handy because Charlie had said that we could meet a black or grizzly bear anywhere on this trail and since I was walking into the wind, neither of us would be aware of the other until we came nose to nose. I had already had enough of bears for one trip, so I was very cautious, and I was aware of how keen my senses had become when expecting the unexpected.

We crossed Wadin Creek, which we had been told would probably be dry. As we crossed through the thick willows that were growing over the creek, we saw that there was a small amount of water running that had formed pools. There was certainly enough for us to have a good drink and refill our water bottles. We remembered Malcolm Groat's advice that many of the creeks in this area might be dry at this time of the year, so we were thankful that this one had some good water running in it. The dogs waded into one of the pools up to their bellies, and lapped the water thankfully, letting the stream wash gently by them, feeling it cooling their hot bodies. The packs got wet, but everything was wrapped in plastic so we weren't worried.

After walking a total of twenty-five kilometres that day, we came to a wide, fast-flowing river, the Red River at last. We dropped our packs on the gravel beach and looked at the clear blue water rushing past, cascading over boulders, swirling around a bend below us and then rushing noisily over the rocks again. It was a picture postcard moment with the green trees framing the boulders over which the bluish-green waters tumbled. Fist-sized rocks, worn smooth, lined the river and the high water mark was evident by the cutbank several metres away.

Charlie announced that this was a very strong river, and we would have to wade across it first thing the next day. I looked at the dogs, and at Antoine, who was half-blind, and thought about my inexperience in these situations. I turned and started to look for a campsite and left thoughts and doubts about crossing this river until tomorrow. Charlie took his rifle and went looking for some game so the dogs could have a good meal.

As we got the camp into shape, we heard a rifle shot but when Charlie came back, he didn't have anything. He said that he had just seen the biggest beaver ever. At first he thought that it was a small bear, but he found where it had been gnawing at a tree. The light was fading when he aimed at the beaver, and if we had not been short of food, he would not have attempted the shot. I could see that he was disappointed, but Antoine was quite philosophical. "Maybe tomorrow," he said.

We were getting to an area that was supposed to be inundated with game animals, but apart from lots of tracks we had seen nothing. The fact that we were sometimes talking or that we had dogs with us may have made a difference or perhaps it was the time of the year when animals moved to a different area. A couple of years after we had been through this area, another Native man came across a large herd of elk there and, after shooting a small one, had more than enough fresh food for his stay.

The sound of the rushing Red River was very pleasing after a day of thirst, and because there was an abundance of the wet stuff, I took the opportunity to wash my clothes and to strip off and have a really refreshing wash in the frigid water. I strung a line and hung up my wet clothes, and then went over to the campfire, where Annie was cooking up a huge bannock in a large frying pan. She made one and then another, and the smell made my mouth water. She told me that I would have to wait, because this bannock was for the dogs. When there were enough of them cooked, I helped to carry them over to where the dogs were tied and watched them eat. I was surprised that they didn't just gobble them up, but ate slowly. I thought that perhaps their stomachs had shrunk or that they were very tired and still thirsty. We took them to the river where they lapped up some water, but they didn't seem excessively thirsty.

The sun set behind some clouds and I felt a few drops of rain—just what I needed when my wet clothes were still hanging

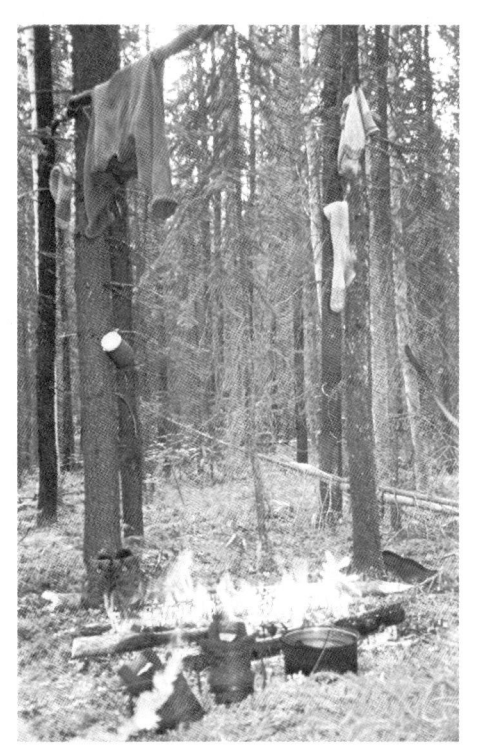

In a moment of respite from the rain, the hikers hang laundry over the campfire.

up. As the light faded, the rain came down more heavily and the mosquitoes and blackflies woke up. They became very pestilent, so we retired to our respective shelters. I felt chilled, and was still suffering from some slight gastrointestinal problems, but I was exhausted too, so my chills were probably from that combination. I got into my sleeping bag and within minutes my problems dissolved in sleep.

Crossing the Red River

By morning, the rain had passed, leaving everything wet and glistening, including the clothes hanging on the line. I felt refreshed after a good night's sleep and when we had eaten our usual breakfast of cereal, which, quite aptly and coincidentally, was a pot of Red River cereal, Charlie went to cut some poles that we were to use to counteract the strong current when we crossed the river. We packed up our camp, but left the dog packs piled up by the side of the river.

Charlie had investigated and found the best place to cross. The water was running fast, but looked to be less than a metre deep, although we would have to negotiate the slippery rocks. Just below us, the water cascaded over rocks. I thought that if we were swept down into them, it would be quite dangerous. In spite of this, I couldn't help but be impressed by the natural beauty before me.

Charlie crossed over first, using a pole to counteract the force of the current. I followed him carrying my pack, leaving the waist strap unfastened in case I slipped. I didn't want to be dragged under. Charlie instructed me on how to brace myself against the current by jamming my pole on the rocky bottom on the downstream side of the current before taking a step. I was going to use a pair of reef shoes that I had brought along for just such an event, but by the time we had walked to the crossing point from our camp, my feet were soaked through so I walked into the water as I was, wearing my rain pants tucked into my socks to try and keep most of my pants dry. The water still found its way up my legs almost to my waist, but that was the least of my worries as I concentrated on keeping my balance.

The rocks were slippery, but using the bracing poles we reached the other side without incident. I dropped my pack on some brush that I had quickly grabbed from the underside of a spruce tree and then waded back into the water to bring some of the dog packs over. Because of Antoine's poor eyesight, Charlie crossed with him to guide him through the calmest waters.

Although Antoine was classified as legally blind, he was one of the best bush men in Fort Ware, living most of his life with Annie in one or the other of their neat cabins north of the village. He trapped for a living in the wintertime, and climbed mountains with Annie as they searched for marmot or mountain sheep, and they were never without meat for long. Antoine was always busy around our camp, cutting and splitting firewood or getting water. He and Annie had been as good as their word about not drinking and I was very impressed with their expert camp skills, carried out in a casual way that made it look almost effortless. Their hiking too was expert, and after a long day on the trail, they never complained of being tired. In many ways, they were the embodiment of the "People of the Rocks."

Annie crossed the Red River without any difficulty, carrying Tiny tucked into her windbreaker, from where she could view the excitement from a warm, dry refuge. I made another trip with Charlie to get the rest of the dog packs.

The dogs had been left loose on the north side of the river. When we had everything all together on the opposite side, Antoine called to his dogs, who ran barking up and down the shore. Finally Boney, the oldest and biggest dog, jumped into the water, and paddling furiously, was swept quickly downstream until he managed to reach the far side farther down and before being swept into the rocks. He dragged himself ashore and shook himself vigorously before bounding up to Antoine, his tail wagging furiously to celebrate the reunion.

We had been so busy watching Boney that we hadn't noticed that as soon as he was halfway across, the other dogs all bounded into the water in a follow-the-leader movement, though they were soon separated in the river and came ashore at different points. When they landed, they were all wet and bedraggled. After shaking themselves vigorously, sending a shower of sparkling water into the surrounding bush, they set about trying to lick themselves dry.

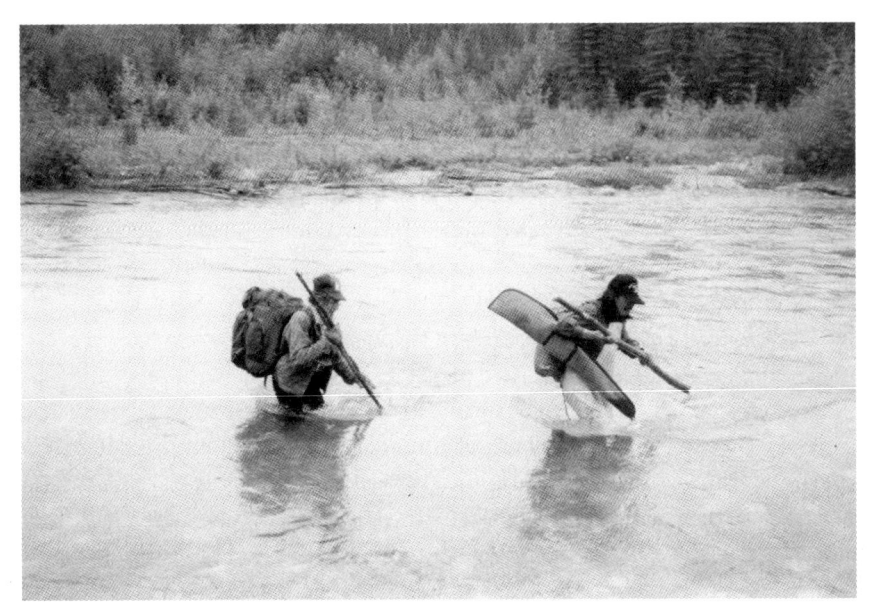

Antoine and Charlie cross the Red River.

We cut down a few small, dry trees and used spruce branches to start a big fire to dry ourselves, and although we had only had breakfast an hour ago, we made some hot tea. The water had been icy cold and it really chilled us, but the fire soon warmed and half dried us. I put on some dry socks, which felt better, but I still had to wear my wet footwear, which was now stiff as well as wet.

All morning we walked through deep wet moss, long grass and puddles of water. The beavers had been very busy all over this part of the country and we came to one flooded area after another. There were a few spots of rain, but I was already soaking wet underneath my rain gear. My legs were sore, my feet were sore, and my back ached, but I had to admit that in some weird sort of way, I was enjoying myself!

Several times when I was feeling a bit uncomfortable, I thought of Old Davie, who would have had to shepherd his large family over these swamps and rivers. Where we had modern equipment and clothing, he had time on his side and his travel schedule must have been quite flexible.

When I was walking behind the others, Bruno, one of Charlie's pack dogs, would look back at me inquiringly, then wait at the side of the trail until I had passed, and then he would walk behind me. This made me feel quite comfortable, because it is very hard to keep glancing behind you when

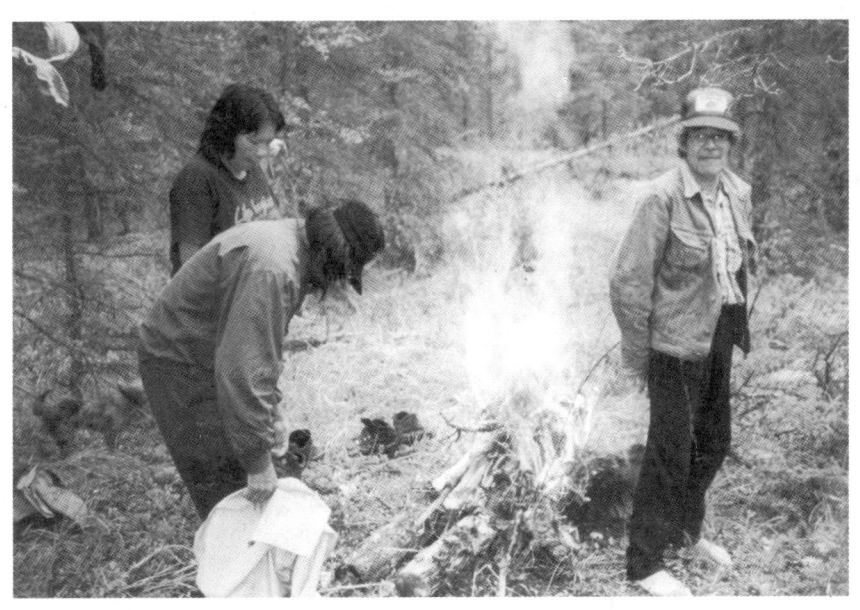

Annie, Charlie and Antoine dry out after crossing the Red River.

you are carrying a large pack, while at the same time trying to anticipate trees jumping out and tripping you up. I was still paranoid about bears, or anything else, coming up behind me, so Bruno became a very good friend. In return, I helped him over or under blowdown trees when he misjudged the height, and wedged himself and his pack under the tree, or found it too high to jump over with his heavy burden. I felt that we had a good symbiotic relationship.

Bad Memories

Airplane Lake is a long, wide lake. The name is clearly printed on the map, but Charlie called it Islands Lake because it has two small islands on the south end and "because we always called it that before those American people crashed their plane near here." For a while we followed a rolling trail through the pine trees down the east side of the lake, until we suddenly came to a broken-down log cabin. It had been built in a small clearing that had an unobstructed view of the lake. The two small islands could be seen farther down and low hills surrounded the rippling waters of this scenic lake. Small bushes were beginning to reclaim the clearing, but the remains of the cabin were plainly visible.

Charlie was unusually quiet, then told us that this was his father's old cabin, where he himself had lived as a young boy, helping his father to trap, fetching water from the lake for his mother, and, I suppose, teasing his sisters. Then one day a plane suddenly arrived unannounced with the Indian Agent along with the RCMP, to enforce a law made by politicians far away, who after a day of work, went home to their spouses and children. For the Boya family, it meant instant breakup of the family unit. Charlie was taken away, along with his brother Willie and his young sisters, to attend the Residential School in Lower Post.

Bad Memories 121

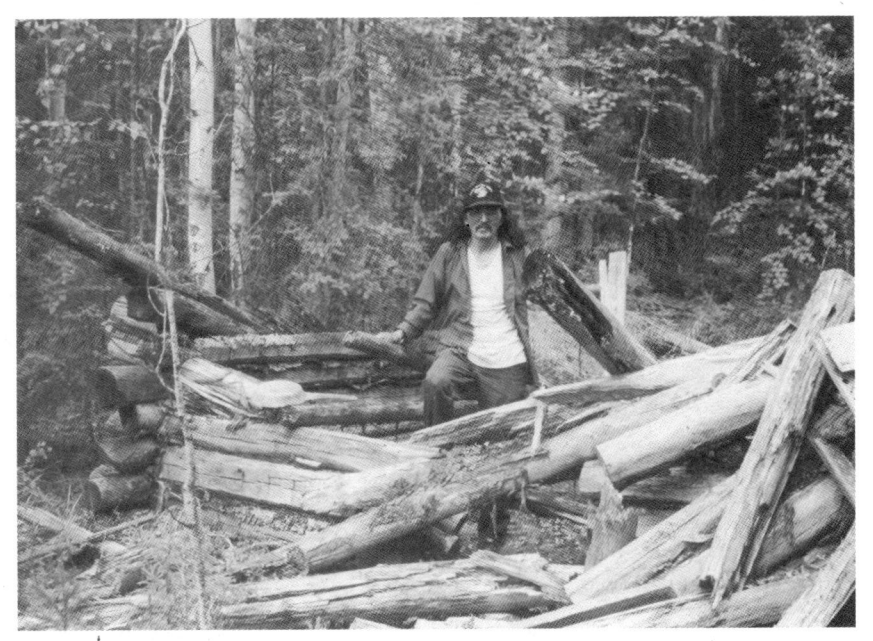

Charlie Boya stands in the wreckage of his boyhood home.

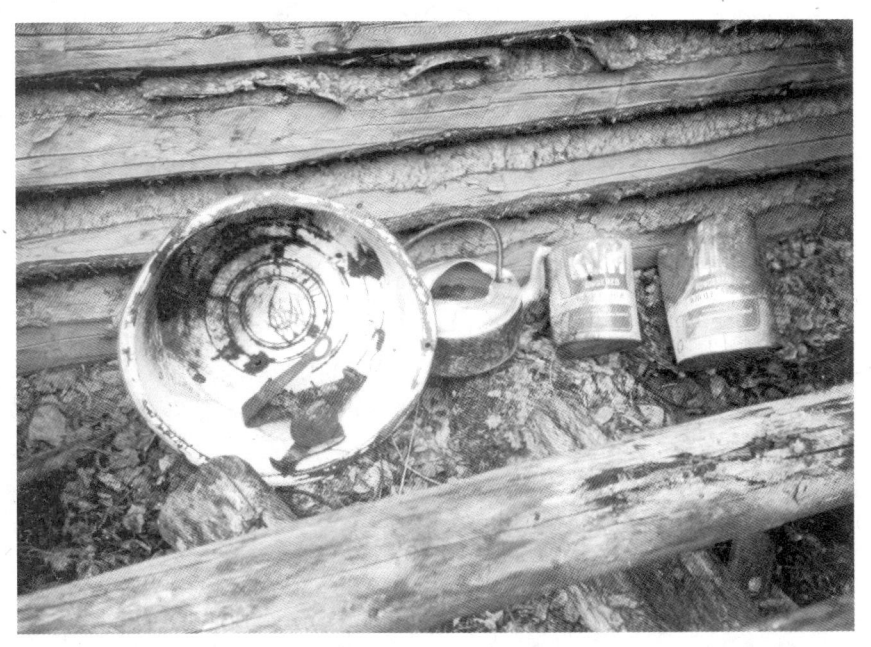

Some artifacts from the Boya cabin: a bowl, a kettle and two tins of Klim milk powder.

Vera, one of Charlie's sisters, told me she was only five years old when they were all taken away from their parents. She stayed at the Residential School for the next twelve years. She also told me later that when she was put on the plane at the cabin, she screamed all the way to Watson Lake. Having three children of my own, I can vividly imagine the devastated feelings of the parents and the fear the children felt when they were taken away. I looked at the cabin and in my imagination I could picture the scene and feel their anguish.

Pieces of an old sled were propped up against a broken-down wall, a sled very similar to the one we had found a long way back on the trail. Charlie rooted around and found an old trap, a kettle, a bowl, and two empty cans of "Klim" milk powder, a staple food item throughout northern Canada in the days of the Hudson's Bay Company and "rations."

Obviously taken back in time, Charlie wandered around, staring at the cabin. Maybe in his mind he was seeing it as it had been when he was a boy and thinking of his now-deceased father, Louis. I looked around too and could picture young Charlie running around in the trees. His father would have surely missed his young industrious son when he was taken away. The girls, too, would have been a great help to the family as they learned how to live in the bush. As the plane left, carrying them all away, the quietness that would have descended must have been heartbreaking. No squeals of laughter, no running around, just silence as the parents wondered what would become of their young ones.

Suddenly Charlie said that we should all move on. I think the memories were upsetting to him. He called to Bruno and set off along the trail again and walked for about an hour before stopping for a tea break. I had favoured camping by the lake but Charlie advised that we had a big hill to climb and it would be better to have that behind us when we camped, rather than face it first thing in the morning. I agreed, but later on, halfway up the hill and out of breath and out of almost everything else, I wondered if I would even make it to the top before breakfast.

Charlie was right. We came to the top, and sure, I was a bit slow, but once I reached the top of the bluff where the camp was already being built by Antoine, I felt the refreshing cool breeze. I could see a large meadow below us with two small lakes at each end. It was the sort of grassy meadow where you could expect to see a moose make an appearance at any time.

The hill was covered with long, coarse grass through which a few hardy bushes grew, along with prickly wild rose bushes that I trampled down so that I could put up my shelter. I hung some of my damp clothes on a line and draped others over the bushes. At the elevation that we were at, the sun seemed to stay high instead of disappearing into the trees as it had in previous camps, and the sun, along with the light breeze, soon dried my clothes. I hoped that the rain would stay away so that we would have a dry day's travel the next day. The sky was clear except for a few wispy clouds over the mountains, and we sat around the campfire talking and watched the sky turn from a ruddy glow to a very deep blue on the horizon.

We talked about Airplane Lake and Louis Boya's cabin, and what it was like to hunt and trap in this location. This led to a discussion about how white men had come into the land, ignoring the people whose land it was, and renamed lakes and mountains that already had names. This was still occurring today when logging and mining companies built roads into isolated areas, supposedly "opening up the country," unaware or ignoring the fact that the country that they were entering had been used for centuries by the original inhabitants. Only a few miles from Fort Ware, for example, there is a small lake that has been used by the village residents for many, many years. A fluorescent blue sign by the side of the road now informs people that its name is Foot Lake, supposedly because it has the shape of a foot. There was no consultation with the Band about the name, even though they had always referred to it in their own language as "Pine Lake." Another sore point with Charlie was how some people, including the press, spoke about them, the Native people, as though they were something to be ignored, or just taken for granted.

Charlie started to talk about his father again and told us how the people who had crashed their plane not too far from Louis' cabin were rescued, and how his father and his friend were not properly acknowledged for the help that they had given.

Plane Crash Survivors

On February 4, 1963, Ralph Flores and Helen Klaben were flying from Whitehorse to Fort St. John in a small plane when they hit a snowstorm. They tried to find the Alaska Highway so that they could follow it down to Fort St. John or return and land at Watson Lake. They had apparently been flying on course—certainly they were following their flight plan that would have taken them to their destination—but when the snow hit, they were quite a long way to the west of the Alaska Highway. Flying lower and lower because of poor visibility, they crashed into trees on the brow of a hill about six kilometres from Airplane Lake.

Both pilot and passenger were seriously injured in the crash. The pilot, Ralph Flores, had a fractured jaw and cracked ribs, and Helen Klaben, the passenger, had a broken arm and a crushed foot. In spite of the injuries, they were able to make a crude shelter. They had very little food with them and it seems they were poorly equipped for flying in isolated areas in winter conditions. Search planes scoured the area without success, and two weeks later the search was called off.

The two survivors lived for forty-nine days through temperatures that dropped to forty below zero, existing on melted snow, a few tins of sardines, two cans of tuna, some fruit cocktail and crackers. Charlie said that he had heard that they also ate a tube of toothpaste.

The victims heard the noise of a chainsaw in the distance and, thinking that it was perhaps a logging camp, they resolved to try to locate the source of the sound when they were physically able to do so. Klaben could not move because of her crushed foot, so after a month of lying helpless in the camp, Flores fashioned some makeshift snowshoes and set off in the direction of the noise.

According to Klaben, in her book, *Hey, I'm Alive!*, Flores managed to get down to a large beaver pond. He walked out onto the lake on his snowshoes and tramped out an SOS with an arrow pointing towards the camp where Klaben lay waiting. After a period of rest, he continued in the direction of the noise that he and Klaben had heard, and then rested again in a makeshift camp. It had taken him four days to reach the pond.

On March 26, 1963, forty-nine days after the plane crash and while Klaben lay at the crash site camp, a plane came over and circled around, having seen the SOS on the lake. Flores was able to signal to the plane with a mirror. The plane landed on Islands Lake, and taxied up to Louis Boya's cabin and alerted Louis and Charlie Porter to the SOS and their sighting of a man, and asked them to go and bring the person back to the cabin. Since it was getting dark, the pilot had to return to base.

Everyone eventually ended up at Louis' cabin, which Klaben described enthusiastically: "It was a lovely log cabin just like the one I imagined living in with my Alaskan husky." They were fed "delicious" moose steaks and "the tea was the best I ever drank."

Louis told Charlie that it was he and his partner, Charlie Porter, "the two Indian trappers" of Klaben's book, who saved the lives of Flores and Klaben by going up to their camps and bringing them to the cabin with a dog sled. In a newspaper story, and in Klaben's book, it says that a pilot found them after seeing an SOS sign in the snow, and alerted the authorities. More planes flew into the area, and one of the pilots had "mushed" up to the crash victims' camp.

When I read the story, I did wonder how a pilot could "mush" anywhere without a dog team. Had he borrowed Louis' team? Or did he send Louis to the camp? Charlie Boya was convinced that in the usual white man's way, they wanted to get all the credit for the rescue for themselves, and as usual, he said that the Natives were just incidental. Another part of the story Charlie objected to was the account of when the pilot first spotted Klaben's camp and he was reported as saying that he saw "maybe an Indian squaw," as though a Native woman would be of no consequence.

In 1998, members of the pilot's family from the United States went to Whitehorse with the idea of going to the crash site as a tribute to Flores, their father, who had passed away in 1997. After our trip was over, Charlie showed me a newspaper cutting describing the visit, which was reported as being in the southeast Yukon. Neither Charlie nor I ever heard if the party made it to the site, but if they had got lost, I'm sure that it would have been in the news. The fact is that Airplane Lake is in British Columbia, about 250 kilometres south of the Yukon's border town of Watson Lake.

That night as we sat discussing the dangers of flying in the north, and especially in the wintertime, we learned, during a satellite phone call to Fort Ware, that two well-known Catholic priests, Ian McCormick and Brian Ballard, who had both been visiting priests to Fort Ware, had been killed in a plane crash southeast of Prince George.

Scoop Lake

As the mountains became more visible and identifiable, we knew we were getting close to the Kechika River, which is about the halfway point of the Davie Trail. The Kechika River starts high up in the Rocky Mountains and flows very close to Terminus Mountain, where Gary Moore has an outfitters lodge. It then continues to flow north past Scoop Lake, where there is another outfitters camp. These are not the canvas tent and food shacks that a vivid imagination might conjure up for a hunting camp, but well-appointed buildings and services fit for a millionaire. We hoped to camp later on at or near Scoop Lake lodge.

As we trudged along the trail, I began to feel my sixty years. I had lost weight for sure, since my pants were looser around the waist and my belt had to be pulled several notches tighter. In one way I felt very fit. I also felt very tired, and my shoulders and legs ached. Annie, the youngest member of our group was only forty-nine years old, and she cruised along as though she was out for a stroll. Antoine, who was a remarkable sixty-one years old, looked the same as the day we had started, as did Charlie, at forty-six years old. Charlie still spent hours reconnoitering a few kilometres of trail every night, at the same time hoping to find some meat, either the four-footed kind or even the feathered variety.

We had done well so far on dried food supplemented with grouse every few days, and I had taken to drinking lots of orange-flavoured juice with a high sugar content to boost my flagging energy. Many magazines promote walking as the best exercise for the human body and this had proved correct for many of the active Kaska and Sekani people. A diet generally low in fats and sugar is recommended and in Aatse Davie's time, sugar was virtually unknown. An Elder in Fort Ware, Mike Abou, now in his seventies, told me that he did not taste refined sugar until he was a teenager. Now sugar is consumed in large quantities through candy, pop and other sweet drinks, and even tea and coffee have sugar added. As a result, diabetes is a national Aboriginal crisis. Only a few people in Fort Ware and Ingenika have been diagnosed with diabetes but that only shows how far behind the rest of their Aboriginal peers they are in changing to a refined southern diet. Because the old-timers' diet was low in fats, the fat of the animals that they killed was all used and a "fat" animal was something to be desired. To show that we were living in some ways as the old-timers did, we too desired some fat and I thought it would be especially desirable if it came attached to a nice steak!

Early in the morning we were following the trail, which was clearly marked with blazes for the first hour of our travel. Then abruptly, we were left scouting around for any sign of a blaze or ribbon, even a cut tree. By spreading out, one or the other of us would find something to indicate where we should go, perhaps another blaze or a worn part of the trail, or sometimes it was simply by forging ahead, knowing that the trail should not make any sudden changes in direction. For the most part we were right, and found our way, although we had to keep making detours around fallen trees. Then, for a short time, the trail was quite good, keeping to reasonably high ground with a few hills to break any monotony, and staying within the timber.

Although I had not seen very many birds except grouse since we started, I now began to hear more birdsong, grouse calling to their young, chickadees twittering away, and woodpeckers ratatatatting trees with their beaks as they searched for insects. Grouse were still drumming, the dull thumping of their dance building to a crescendo before abruptly stopping. The season was late if they were looking for a mate, so I wondered if they were practising for next year. I caught a glimpse of a yellow warbler hunting for insects amongst the willow and alder branches. We had seen the two swans, loons, and some mallard ducks earlier on, but as the land rose towards the mountains, we seemed to be getting away from large bodies of water and the birds that were attracted to wetlands.

Animal tracks increased as we came to a swampy area, where reeds and grasses grew in profusion. The trail became more trampled down as the tracks converged, as animals came from every direction and headed towards some common goal. Our trail had either disappeared again or had been obliterated by the big ungulates, so we went in the same direction that the animals had taken.

A sulphur smell emanating from a brownish-grey mud had evidently attracted the moose to this highly mineralized area, and they had been there by the dozens. Their hooves had churned up the ground so much that we had difficulty in finding a passage that avoided the sticky mud. We wound our way over the grassy humps and with some relief gained dry ground on the other side where Annie spied an old blaze that confirmed that we were back on the trail.

From the map, we saw that we should have crossed Birches Creek already, and as we sweated along in the blazing sun, we began to think that we had passed it unnoticed. We felt that we should now be almost at the Kechika River, one of our major goals on this section of the trip, but it always seemed to be "over the next rise." We descended a steep bank and found ourselves looking at a fast-running creek: Birches Creek.

The creek was knee-deep and about four metres wide. It was clear and inviting, and we drank our fill of the cold water, filling our bottles in case this was the last good source of fresh water. Even Antoine took a long drink of the water, which he rarely drank during the day; instead he filled up with countless cups of tea every time we made a campfire. Antoine removed the dog packs from the dogs and he and Annie waded across with some of the packs after shedding boots and socks. I also carried some packs over and Charlie carried Bruno over, dog pack still attached.

The trail led down to the creek where, to our surprise, we found a large piece of painted plywood lying in the bush. Here we were in the middle of the wilderness miles from anywhere and we come across this symbol of human technology! The plywood may have fallen off a pack-horse, but there was no sign of horses in the area. Nearby was a moose skull with the antlers still attached, but it is doubtful that the skull would have been left by any hunters, because they were quite an impressive size and would have been taken along for brag value. Our curiosity was not satisfied.

Once we had crossed the creek and repacked the dogs again, we hoisted our own packs and set off up the bank only to find that the trail was nowhere to be found. Not a blaze, ribbon, cut branch, nothing. We went back to where the trail had come out at Birches Creek and looked to see where the trail should have logically gone.

After about an hour of dodging through the trees, we came to a fast-moving creek again, and, studying the lay of the land along with the map, we concluded that it was Birches Creek again—it was shown as a serpentine creek, winding this way and that, until a long way off, it emptied into the Kechika River. We stopped for a short rest and Annie said that the dry, hot weather was drying out her skin, so she plastered some Nivea cream over her face. I laughed and asked if she was making herself into a white woman. She took this as a good joke and I took a photograph of her coated in the cream.

If the creek had been easy to follow we would probably have used it to take us to the Kechika River, but thick bush on either side of it made it impossible to forge ahead. We walked to higher ground to the south of the creek and as we climbed, we came to a plateau that had suffered a forest fire perhaps ten or fifteen years ago. Scrub bush and closely packed, shoulder-high new-growth pine trees made for difficult walking, compounded by the fallen, blackened trees which lay over the whole area like a game of pick-up sticks.

Several times I stumbled or slipped as I was balancing along a blackened tree spur, and fell head over heels into the underbrush, my pack pushing me down. I was feeling very frustrated at not being able to stay upright when I caught sight of the dogs, their coats and packs flecked with sooty residue, jumping over and squeezing between the deadfall. And I thought I had it tough! Antoine manoeuvred over the trees better than I did, only falling once, and I was chagrined when he had to come and help me extricate myself from between two logs shortly afterwards.

We could see the gap in the land where the Kechika River cut through the plateau, and we resolved to keep going to the river and make camp there. There was no water anywhere through the old burn, so it was no good even thinking of making camp there. We pushed on over the high ground where the new growth of pine trees seemed endless. Looking ahead, I kept thinking that the plateau must surely end just over the horizon—but on and on it went. It was seven-thirty in the evening and twenty-seven kilometres from our last camp when we suddenly came to the plateau's edge. There, from a high ridge, we looked down upon the swift-flowing, wide Kechika River about two kilometres from where we stood.

We sat down, enjoying the cooling breeze, and rested while we watched the river flowing north through a large flat valley where jackpine lay like a huge green carpet over the whole landscape. The Rocky Mountains could

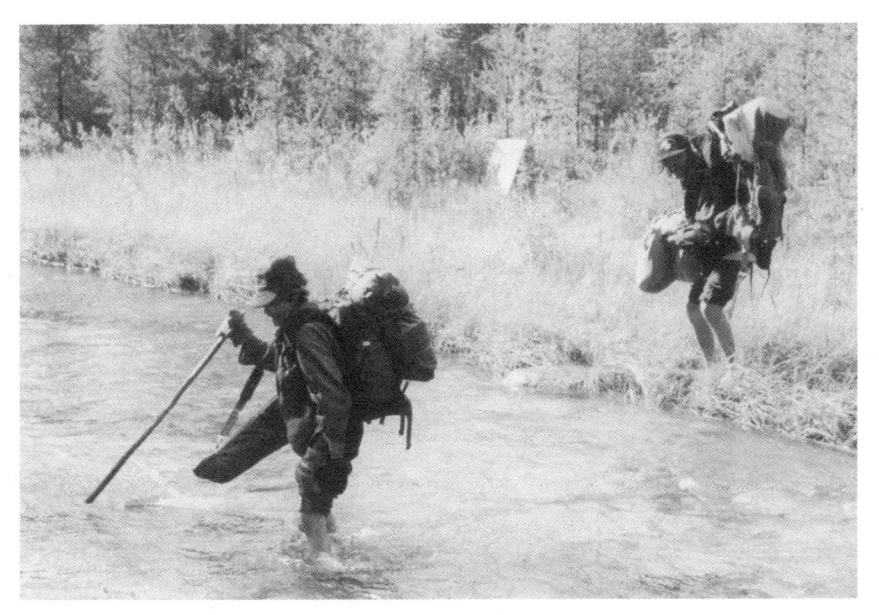

Antoine and Charlie cross Birches Creek.

be seen in the distance to the east, and to the southwest, the Omenica Mountains stood out on the horizon.

We stayed there for about half an hour, mesmerized by the view, thankful that at last we were out of the burned-over land. Then when we got up, feeling stiff and beginning to notice the bite of the cold wind blowing over the ridge, the thought of fresh water and a place to make camp spurred us on. The ridge that we rested on had been used as a lookout and thoroughfare by moose, deer and elk, and their trail followed along the crest. We followed the ridge for a short way, then saw where the animals had slid down the bank, so we followed suit and slipped and scrambled down the shale as they had, to the level ground below, then walked through the mossy bush for another half an hour.

Charlie forced his way through the trees and willows and river flotsam that had been left after last spring's high water and we followed him, spurred on by the knowledge that we would rest in a few minutes. I heard Charlie shout triumphantly as he came out onto the rocky shore of the Kechika and as soon as we joined him, we divested ourselves of our packs. After taking a long drink of Kechika water, we cleared a small flat area on the bank of the river and made camp in some willow bushes, two old fallen trees marking a comfortable room for us to sit in while we ate macaroni and vegetable soup.

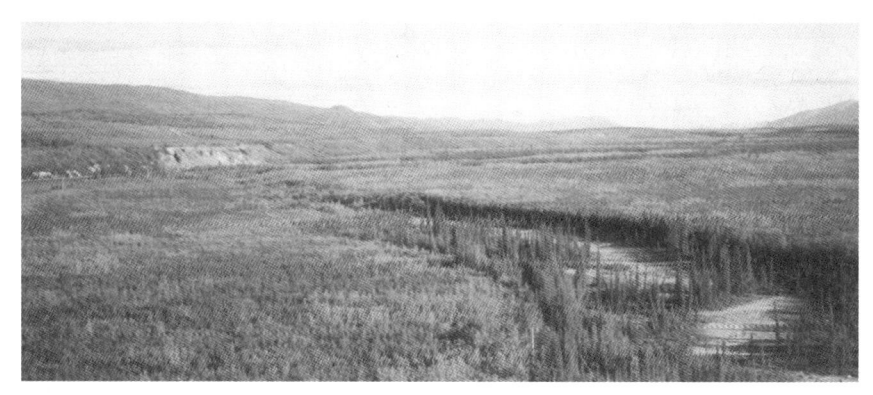

At last, the hikers catch sight of the Kechika River.

I drank several mugs of tea, a bottle of water and, to top it off, I mixed some powdered milk with water.

As we sat around talking in the fading light, dancing shadows jumping over us from the flames of the campfire, I could not help but think how our roles had evolved, perhaps by design, perhaps for comfort. Charlie, of course, has been the guide, and Annie emerged as a support trail-finder when we were moving. Then she became the camp cook when camp was made at the end of the day. Antoine, on the other hand, had been the dog master, expertly fastening the dog packs. I never saw any of his dogs needing to have their pack readjusted during the day. He was also expert at camp construction and maintenance and was always the one who had a fire blazing away within minutes of us stopping, rain or shine. My role? Most of the time it seemed I just tried not to get in the way, but I was able to gather some dry firewood, get water, and put up my shelter and keep a record of our progress. It was obvious that my three travel companions were comfortable anywhere in the bush and could make a cozy camp as easily as I could make my bed at home. I felt very relaxed in their presence.

As night fell and the conversation lagged, I took myself to the shelter that I had constructed by the side of the river, crawled thankfully into my sleeping bag, and slept through the night. When I woke up and looked out through the mosquito netting, I saw the river blanketed in swirling mist. When I checked the temperature on my mini-thermometer, I saw that it was only a few degrees above zero. I had a drink and waited for the sun to rise.

The sun eventually rose over the Kechika, its rays sparkling in the river mist. I lay in my shelter and surveyed the swirling mists. They looked like an Impressionist painting as the sun was reflected in the water molecules, which then danced in a rainbow of colour. It was so fascinating, I didn't want to get up.

I set my solar charger and satellite phone in the sun when the mists had burned off. While we ate breakfast, we talked about building a raft to cross the wide Kechika, a river that was four or five times as wide as the Red River we had crossed earlier. The current here was much stronger and flowing very fast in the direction opposite to the one we were going. If we did not paddle hard enough, and were carried downstream by the current before we could land, it would add many more kilometres to our travels—something we were not at all keen to have happen. With the four of us and the dogs and all our packs, we would have to either make two crossings with a raft, or build a large unwieldy craft that would be too difficult to paddle. There were no cottonwood trees in this part of the country and when we looked around, there were no dry pine or spruce trees that were large enough for our purpose.

According to the Kaska map, the trail followed a height of land to the west of the Kechika, although we had found no sign of it. Charlie was aware of a trail on the east side of the Kechika. It was shown on one of our maps and he had been on that trail a few years ago when he had been hunting north from his cabin at Terminus Mountain, but he had never had to cross this section of the river. Trying to think what Aatse Davie would have done or what the horse and mule packers would have done did not help us to find a solution. There was a creek almost opposite to where we were camped on the Kechika that was appropriately called Boya Creek. It flowed from a

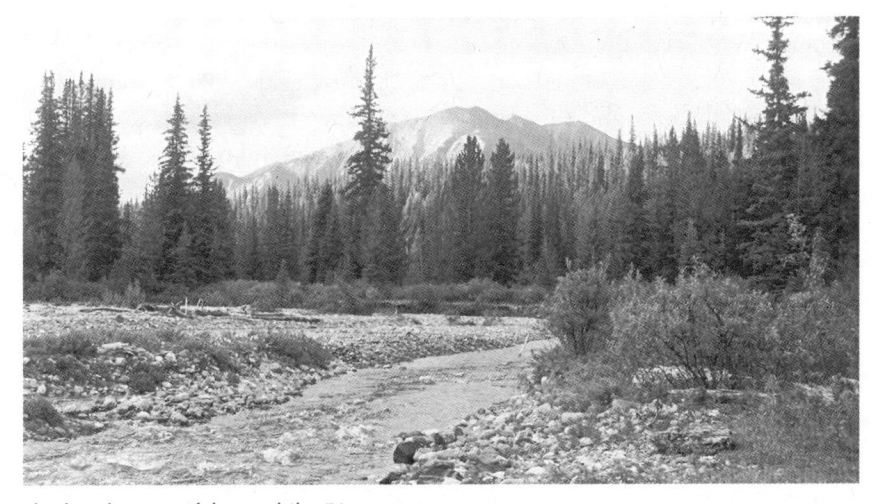

The headwaters of the Kechika River.

northeasterly direction and drained into the Kechika from Graveyard Lake. The Kaska map said that the eastern trail was "only inferred."

We were running short of food, though we could have managed another few days, but the dogs had not had a real meal for three days and were surviving on scraps. Charlie shot a squirrel and gave it to Boney, who ate it within seconds. The other dogs looked dejected when they didn't get any.

We had a long discussion about flying to Scoop Lake rather than continuing the trek on foot. With the uncertainty of finding a good trail and having to cross the wide Kechika twice, at this stage of the exercise, I felt that flying held a certain charm. Tradition and cultural experiences were put aside in favour of a modern and more practical form of transportation though each of us felt disappointed at the prospect of finishing our hike short of the halfway goal. It almost felt like cheating.

I put in a phone call to Randy Gee, a pilot from Fort St. John who had a business interest in one of the lodges on the Kechika and consequently flew into the area quite frequently. After explaining our situation and location to him, he agreed to come and pick us up and take us the short distance to Scoop Lake. Some time later a small plane flew overhead, circled and taxied onto the river, but it wasn't Randy piloting the plane, it was Darwin Cary. He was on his way north to Watson Lake. Randy had called him from Fort St. John and found that Darwin could manage to move us with his plane, so Darwin had dropped by to tell us that he was planning to pick us up on his return journey to Scoop Lake.

As we waited for Darwin to return, Antoine, Annie and Charlie walked up the river to see if there was any game, and saw nothing but tracks. When they returned, we ate a lunch of soup and bannock, and as we were finishing, we heard the sound of a boat heading downriver towards us. A large, noisy jet-powered river boat came into view with several men on board. We waved, but they didn't even look our way, and soon they were lost to view downriver. We sat back again to wait. If we had been insistent on crossing the river, we would have jumped up and down and fired the rifle in the air and made much more of a fuss to get their attention, then perhaps we would have had an easy, dry way over.

Eventually Darwin arrived and landed with his float plane and we loaded our supplies and equipment, passing everything from the rocky shore to Darwin who stood carefully on a pontoon as he stowed the packs. We even lifted the dogs over so that they would not get wet and consequently wet us and everything else that was on the plane. Once in the plane, the dogs sat quietly as though they were quite content to let someone else do the work.

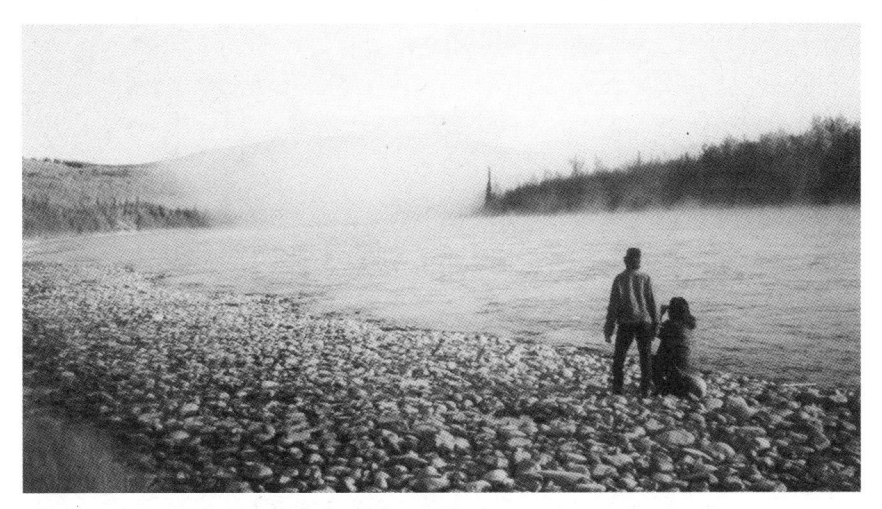

Antoine and Annie at the bank of the Kechika River.

We arrived at Scoop Lake, the plane skimming over the calm waters of the small lake and within minutes of taxiing to the dock, we were unloading all the supplies. We walked towards the lodge, passing a sign that read "Scoop Lake Outfitters welcomes you to the Rocky Mountain Trench, 'Seventh Wonder of the World,' Gateway to Trophy Hunting and Fishing." We had been quite prepared to camp, but Darwin had already made preparations for us to stay in a couple of his bunkhouses. Charlie and I took one and Antoine and Annie took the one next to us.

The dogs were tied up a little way from the cabins so that they would not get into an argument with Darwin's dogs, which ran around loose. The hungry dogs were then fed a good meal, supplied by Donna, Darwin's wife.

Darwin showed us around his property, and we looked at the lodge and the cabins, which were all built of logs. He reserved an outbuilding for preparing the hunter's trophies. I was very impressed with the size of some wolf pelts that were in one of his cabins. I thought that I had seen large wolves before, but never anything as large as those that inhabited the Trench. The largest was at least three metres long from nose to tail, and the animal must have weighed close to forty-five kilograms. Darwin explained that a pack of six to eight wolves needed at least one moose or several deer or an elk every week just to keep them from starving. We looked with awe at the ingenious computerized solar system that he had constructed and which provided most of the power for the lodge in the summertime.

We were invited into the main cabin for a huge meal of stew and pasta, with lemon juice to drink. Then, as we were served lovely fresh coffee, Mrs.

136   Tse-loh-ne

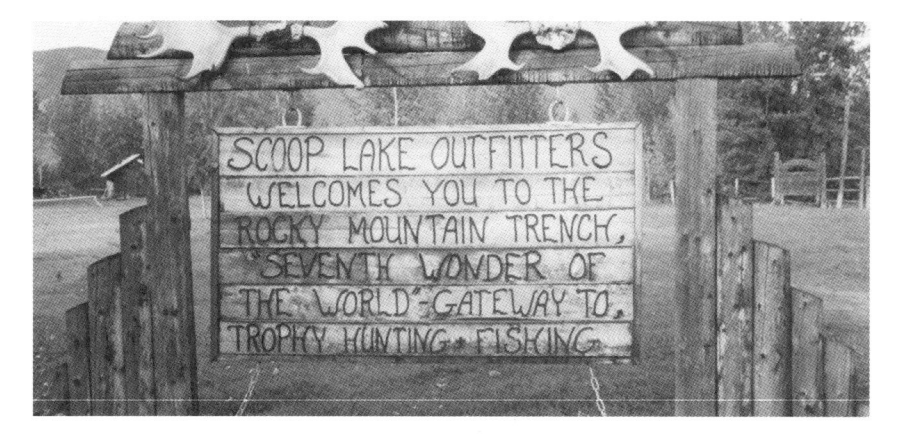

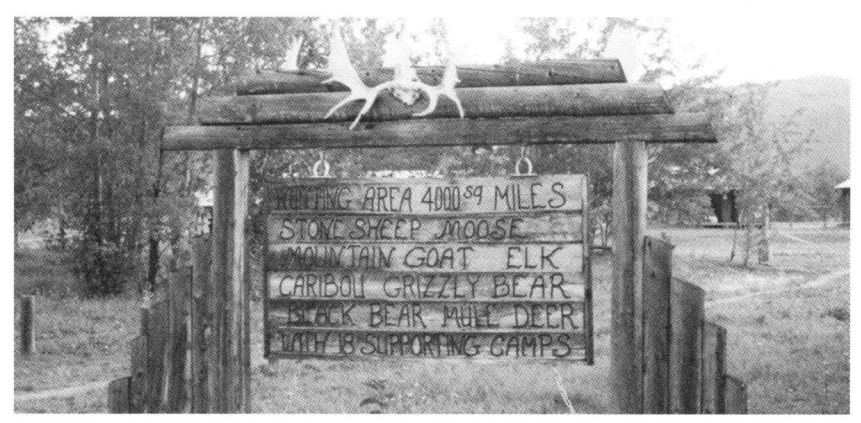

Top: Scoop Lake Outfitters welcome visitors to the "Seventh Wonder of the Wold."
Bottom: The Serengeti of the North boasts a variety of prey for hunters.

Cary brought out some sweet cake with a chocolate topping. We sat around a comfortable sitting room and swapped stories about living in the bush. I thought about Aatse Davie and the Kaska and Sekani of old who never enjoyed a warm and comfortable bed anywhere on their travels through this hard country.

Antoine and Annie were to fly home to Fort Ware with their dogs the following day. They had been such good friends and we had forged a lasting bond. It was good to sit with them and listen to their stories. Before we separated, we discussed the trip. Like any adventure we were inclined to talk about the positive things, the unknowns, the good experiences and the camaraderie that we had shared. We also felt that we should talk about the shortcomings of the trip, like the poor trail through the swamps, the neglect

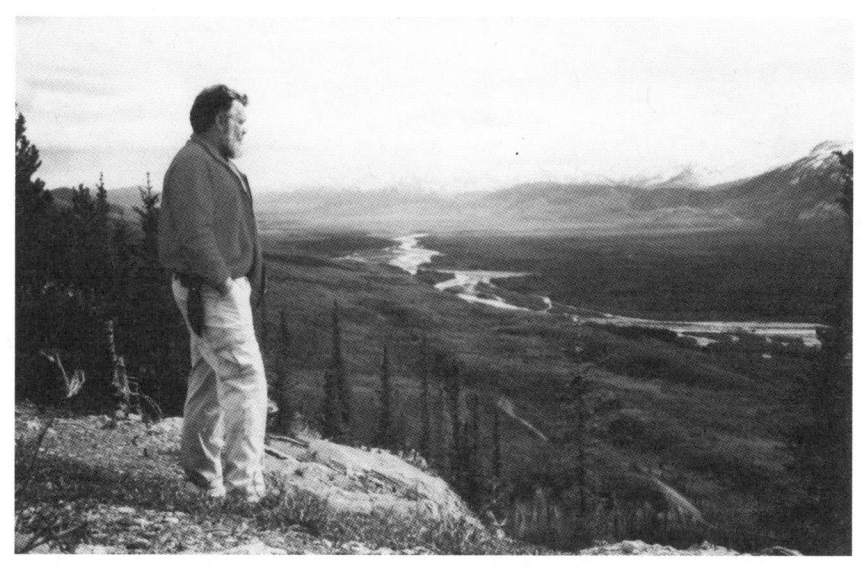

The author views the Kechika River in the Rocky Mountain Trench.

of cabins like Louis Boya's, and the difficulty of crossing the Kechika River. Antoine and Annie were eager to go home where they would hunt for a winter's supply of meat and put up the important wood supply at their cabin at Twelve Mile. We were very aware of our own problems that sometimes made it impossible for us to follow our dreams.

As we sat talking in the warm room, I became conscious of the smell of smoke and spruce needles that seemed to emanate from us. In camp it had seemed quite normal, but now I knew that it was something that our hosts did not share. Perhaps they were too polite to comment, so I thought maybe I should mention that I had become aware of a lack of personal freshness so that our hosts would not have to be the first to suggest that we take a shower. Consequently, we were invited to take long, hot showers. Fortunately our hosts were used to hunters coming into the cabin after days out in the bush so a certain lack of personal freshness was something they expected from their clients!

As I stood under the blast of hot water, many of the aches and pains seemed to follow the water down the drain. Feeling warm, clean and very sleepy, I went to the bunkhouse. I climbed into my smoky sleeping bag, and using a luxuriously soft pillow that was in the cabin, I sank into a very deep sleep thinking about this unique and wild country.

John Ogilvie "Skookum" Davidson

For the next section of trail that led from Terminus Mountain to Fort Ware, the Kaska Tribal Council had contracted with Eric Gunderson from North West Environmental Group Ltd. in Williams Lake to identify strategic points along the way using a Global Positioning System (GPS). He was also to identify places where the trail might need to be relocated because of newly formed beaver ponds, a problem that was a direct result of the lack of trappers and the resulting proliferation of beaver. Another problem was that over the years the river had relocated itself during many spring thaws with its raging seasonal rivers. The team was also to make recommendations for the possible placement of basic log cabins that could be built for future tourist use. On this section of the trail, Jason Harris, a young graduate student from the University of Calgary, was to identify and document gravesites and any other archaeological or historical discoveries that were found along the way. Charlie Boya was going to guide us, since this was territory that he was very familiar with. Eric Gunderson would write a report for the Kaska Tribal Council once we reached the end of the trail. Charlie's wife, Hazel, was going to join us for this section of the hike and act as cook. Antoine and Annie Charlie were going into the mountains to hunt sheep.

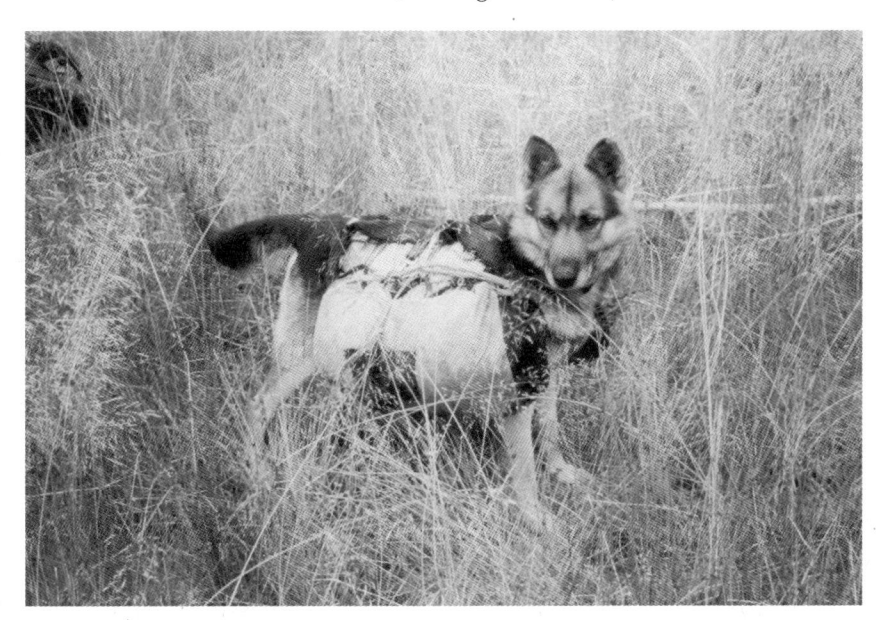

Pack dog Bruno.

To add to the party, Charlie was going to bring three of his pack dogs. They were needed to help pack supplies since we would no longer have Antoine's sturdy dogs to pack for us. This fitted in nicely with our continued focus on tradition—the Kaska and Sekani had used pack dogs for over a hundred years whenever they moved camp or went hunting.

Bruno, a well-trained dog, would continue with us down the trail. Tyson was a new dog of no particular breed, but he had that floppy-eared, good-natured look about him. Then there was Goldie, who looked like a cross between a golden Lab and a collie, but he could have had all sorts of mixtures in his bloodlines. Goldie had been on a mountain trip packing for Charlie some months before, and had fallen down a cliff, dislocating his shoulder, but had apparently made a good recovery. We were hoping so anyway!

Unlike Old Davie and his family, we had a few days' respite and a quick visit to Fort Ware to replenish our supplies. I flew back to the trail from Fort Ware on a small plane that was going to pick up a young student from a Kaska Rediscovery Wilderness camp. I arrived at Terminus Mountain early in the morning on a clear sunny day. Charlie, Hazel, Eric and Jason were to fly up to meet me at outfitter Gary Moore's hunting lodge the following day. Wild animals abound at Terminus Mountain, and Gary owns and manages the lodge, flying his own plane, bringing in hunters who come from all over the world to see this famous section of the "Serengeti of the North." It was refreshing to see wild animals grazing in close to the lodge and I couldn't help wondering where all the animals had been north of Scoop Lake and Terminus Mountain. There would now be no shortage of food in the Terminus Mountain area, or so I thought.

Like the lodge at Scoop Lake, the lodge here was built of logs and so were the cabins. Everything was laid out neatly. An old greying barn and a few other relics from Skook Davidson's Diamond J Ranch days were still in evidence although Gary Moore plans to refurbish the whole site eventually. The lodge sits in a clearing where the grass is kept cut, just like a lawn. A gravel airstrip is about half a kilometre down a dirt trail and at the end of the strip is a large hay meadow.

In winter, warm winds often blow through a gap between the Omenica Mountain Range in the southwest and the Cassiar Range to the northwest, and in this area the frozen mountain streams soon become surging rivers early in the springtime. These rivers flood the low-lying earth, watering the rich ground, which in turn nourishes an abundance of deciduous trees and bushes.

In the springtime, "prescribed burning" is undertaken to encourage new growth of deciduous trees, willow bushes and bunch grass, which of course, the deer, elk and other animals eat. Charlie Boya had been employed in previous years to do the burning by the Game Management Branch and he told of seeing the valley full of smoke after he had set fire to the dry underbrush. It eventually burned itself out, leaving the ground quite undamaged, and as is the case in rural areas where dead grass has been burned, green shoots soon appeared through the blackened ash.

A stone's throw from the main lodge is the base of Terminus Mountain. As I wandered around, I found a trail that led to the high ground just behind one of the barns. I wanted to see for myself if there were as many sheep and goats as the lodge advertised, so I took advantage of the sunny day to climb the mountain.

As I started up on the trail behind the lodge, I saw a memorial plaque set in a rock monument that had been placed there in memory of Skook Davidson. Skook Davidson had come to Terminus Mountain in 1939 as a horse wrangler for Swannell, one of the first government surveyors. At the end of the trip, when the survey had been completed as far as Terminus Mountain, Skook was offered the horses, because it would have been more expensive to have them wrangled all the way back down south. Since the

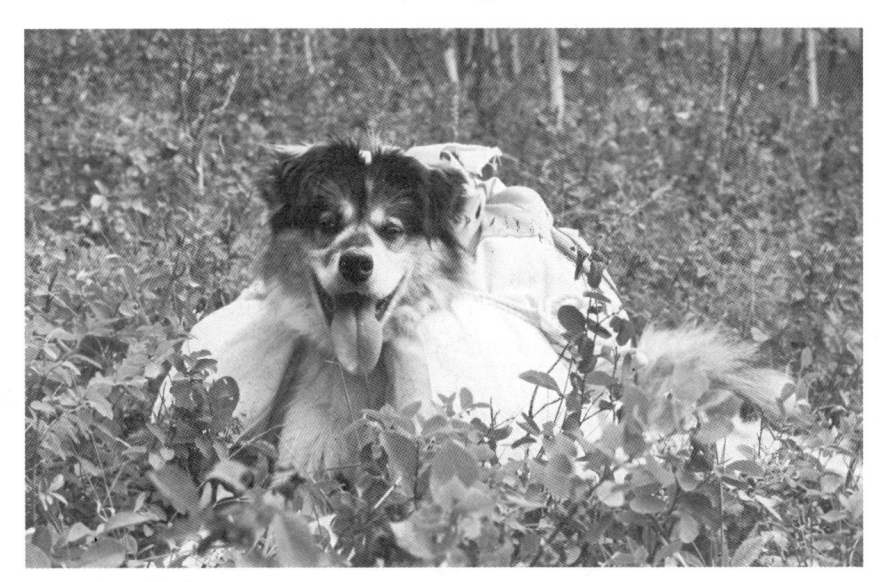

Tyson the pack dog.

area they were in was good for growing feed for livestock, Skook accepted the horses and built himself what he named the "Diamond J Ranch."

Skook reportedly learned to master pack trains as a young man from another famous packer, Cataline. Cataline was the nickname of Jean Jaques Caux, who packed out of Yale, Ashcroft and Hazelton, using as many as sixty "perfectly trained" mules. Later, after working and travelling with Swannell when the northern Interior was being surveyed, Skook ran a thriving business with pack horses, travelling from Smithers to Fort St. James (where he was well known for kicking up quite a storm for as long as his money lasted). From there, he went north to Germansen Landing following the Baldy Road, then turned east over to the Rocky Mountain Trench, to Fort Grahame. He then followed the Davie Trail north to Terminus Mountain, and then from there he went on to Lower Post.

Skook, whose real name was John Ogilvie "Skookum" Davidson, was a crusty old man and Charlie had the doubtful pleasure of working for him when he was still a very young man. He told many tales concerning Skook as we hiked down the trail that Skook himself had hiked with his famous pack horses not too many years previously.

Known widely for his ability to travel long distances with his pack horses, Charlie said that Skook also had other skills. He was an expert at baking bread, and, in general, a very good cook. This fact was not universally known, but the ranch hands were very thankful for this side of the man. Skook may have been a good cook but, according to Charlie, he did not have very much of a culinary imagination.

One day Skook made a huge pot of meat stew and served it day after day after day. Finally Charlie and another ranch hand approached him and asked if on his next grocery order he could maybe order some other vegetables and some fruit, maybe even some mandarin oranges. Skook looked at them in disbelief. "If you don't like my grub you can (expletive, expletive, expletive). Don't you know how much that stuff costs? Now get out of here with your damn fool ideas."

The two young men retired to the bunkhouse, themselves cussing Skook for his pig-headed attitude. Charlie turned on the radio to try to cheer themselves up a bit. It had only been on a few minutes when they heard Skook's VHF radio phone cut into their program. They couldn't believe their ears when they heard Skook talking to Stan, a pilot from Watson Lake: "Oh, and Stan, maybe you could put in a few cases of vegetables and fruit, and, ah, a case of mandarin oranges. You know I like to look after my boys out here." The boys let out a holler of joy and wide grins spread over their faces.

"Come on, let's go over to Skook's," they said, and into Skook's cabin they swaggered, smiling knowingly.

"What the hell you boys grinning at? Nothing to smile about around here, now git!"

They left without telling Skook what they had overheard, but maybe left Skook feeling that his gruff exterior had remained intact.

A number of First Nations young people worked for Skook, feeding the horses and cutting the winter supply of wood. There was a small cabin down on what was known as Cottonwood Flats where the ranch hands usually stayed and where they would haul down sacks of oats to feed the horses.

One winter day, one of Charlie's friends, Roy Abou, had made some homebrew and invited Charlie to go the cabin at the Flats to sample some. They had a few drinks and his friend also had a mickey, which they also drank. They then decided to go and visit Skook. As they were leaving the cabin, Charlie's friend dashed back into the cabin to fill the stove with firewood so it would be warm when he came back. They arrived at the ranch house feeling no pain, and Skook asked them what the devil was the matter with them, were they not well? They made some reply that must have convinced Skook they were indeed unwell, because he told them to go and rest until they felt better.

Eventually they wandered back down to the Flats and as they rounded a corner Charlie stared into the gloom. He thought that the effects of the brew was making things disappear.

"Where the hell is the cabin?" Roy asked.

They both stared. The cabin had disappeared, burned to the ground. All that was left was a pile of smoking ash and some horses standing around hoping to be fed.

They assumed that when the stove was filled up with dry wood that either the lid or the air vent was left open, and sparks and heat had done the rest. They went back to the ranch house. Skook was as mad as a hatter. Charlie was fortunate in that he was staying with Skook at the ranch house but his friend was made to set a tent frame, a canvas tent on a wood foundation, with plywood walls where he lived all through the winter and into the following spring.

A hard-working and hard-drinking man until he was sixty-five, Skook had a woodsman's vocabulary and was even known to curse over the radio phone. He told anyone who objected that if they didn't like it, they could turn the radio off. In an excerpt from the book, *Notes From the Century Before*, Edward Hoagland describes Davidson as "a cranky old man, crippled up with arthritis, cussing into his radio, who gives a report on his wolves instead of his weather, and throws the cork into the creek when he opens a bottle of whiskey so there won't be a way of stopping the fun." He played jokes and had jokes played on him, but he was said to shoot at anyone who really got on the wrong side of him. Charlie saw the soft side of Skook at times, like an occasion when he overheard Skook talking about him: "One thing about Sonny [Charlie], he's a damn fine worker."

Skook was a very accomplished guide and packer, and in a part of the country that was almost untouched by hunters in those days, trophy animals abounded. But although game was plentiful around the ranch, Skook initiated a one-mile "no shooting" zone. If they needed meat, he would send

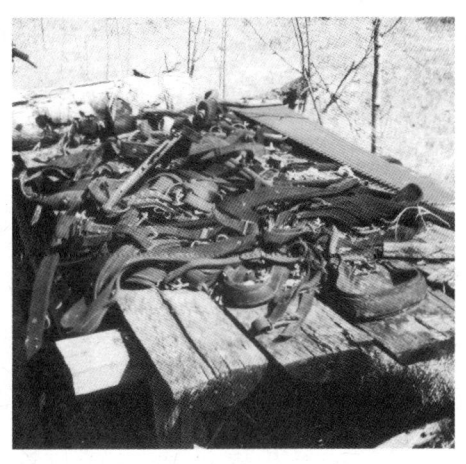

Skook Davidson's harnesses.

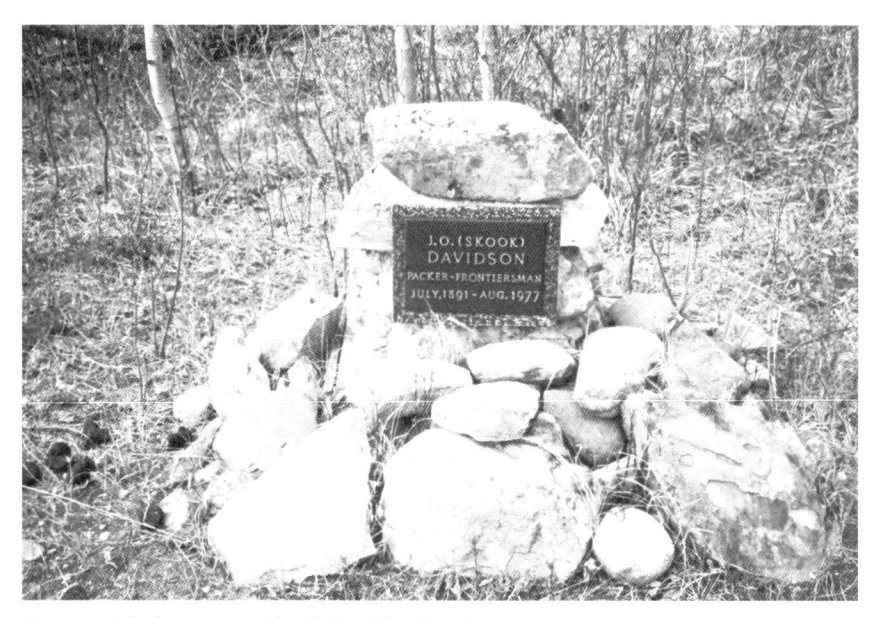

A memorial plaque over Skook Davidson's cairn.

the boys a long way to get it. Of course, the boys being boys, they would go somewhere out of sight, shoot a deer and skin it behind the shack, and cook the meat. Although the boys did not realize it, Skook did let First Nations people get meat in the area because he knew that they would only take what was immediately needed.

On one of these escapades, Charlie and his friend had shot a deer and made a pot of boiled meat. Just as they were feeling satisfied with themselves, they saw Skook walking down towards their cabin with his old dog in tow. They whipped the pot of meat into the wood box, put a lid on the pot and hurriedly threw some firewood on top. Skook came in and they sat around and talked with him, until Skook's dog went into the room where the meat was hidden and a few minutes later, after knocking over the firewood box, the dog walked up to Skook's chair chomping on some ribs he had found in the pot. Skook wanted to know what he had got, and Charlie said that the dog must just have picked up an old bone. "Oh that's okay, just let him chew on that old bone then!" Skook replied. If he knew what was going on he didn't let on, but it sure made Charlie and his friend sweat.

The Davie Trail was worn down about thirty centimetres in places, as though someone had cut a very even, shallow trench. Apparently this was caused by the numerous animals that the old packer Skook mustered through the Trench. This trail phenomena can be seen in many places even now, especially where the land is soft and where wild animals have continued to use this ready-made roadway.

The late Les Bower, a long-time bush pilot for Northern Thunderbird Air, told me that on a stopover at Terminus Mountain, he sat and visited with Skook, who told him that he had a large collection of photographs and diaries in the attic of his old cabin. Les told him that he should make sure that they were safe because of their historical significance, but Skook didn't think it was important and never did anything with them. Years later, when Skook was away from the ranch, the cabin burned down in what Charlie Boya maintained were suspicious circumstances, although he wouldn't elaborate. The photographs and diaries were all burned to cinders, and Les, who loved to listen and tell stories of the old-timers of the north, felt that it was a great loss to British Columbia.

In an overgrown clearing not too far from the lodge, a narrow horse wagon sat in the sunlight, and amongst the accumulated leaves and detritus of the seasons was a tangled mass of black harnesses, dried and brittle, which I was told was all that was left of Skook's outfit. Maybe it still sits there even today in the sun and the snow and the rain, never to be used again in this day of mechanization. Like much outdated horse equipment, it will slowly disintegrate and be lost in the grasses and willows that will spring up around it.

Thirteen kilometres east-northeast of Dall Lake and to the west of Skook's territory sits a permanent tribute to this tough old-timer who died in 1972: Mount Skook Davidson rises 2,382 metres. After his death, Skook's ashes were cast over the valley that he loved so much.

The Turnagain River

I continued my climb up the steep, grassy bank that was being slowly eroded by the wind and the weather, and immediately noticed some movement above me. Almost on cue, four Stone's sheep came out of the trees. They went over to the greyish-white clay and started nibbling at the mineral-rich ground. As I approached them, the sheep moved away cautiously, but they were not too nervous. Later in the day, when I returned to the lodge, Gary told me that the traditional "no shoot" zone that Skook had initiated still applied and that no one was allowed to shoot anything in the vicinity of the lodge. Consequently, the animals had learned that they were safer around the hunting lodge than they were in their normal habitat in the rocks.

I followed a sheep track along a high ridge that fell away to a deep canyon. Halfway across, I became quite aware that I wasn't as surefooted as the animals I had been watching and, with my heart in my mouth, I edged over to where the undergrowth gave me something to hang on to. I wandered around on the mountainside, keeping the lodge in view far below me. I sat down on a rock to catch my breath and enjoyed the gentle breeze that swept up to me from the valley below. The breeze whispered through a small stand of aspen trees, making their leaves tremble. As I sat there I looked down over the valley again and towards the south I could see the Kechika River, its waters glistening in the sunlight as it wound down from the distant mountains. I wondered with a twinge of excitement what it would be like walking along its banks.

In some scree higher up the steep sides of the mountain, I saw some white specks and thought perhaps it was some residual snow from last winter—except the specks didn't stay still. I pulled out my binoculars and counted eight mountain goats, including three kids. I didn't want to risk getting too close so I just stayed where I was, watching them move slowly across the rocks.

Returning to the lodge a little later, I surprised two deer, or more correctly, they surprised me. After they had stared at me for a moment with their big eyes, they suddenly turned and bounced away into the trees as though they had springs in their heels. I crossed in front of the hay barn and saw two of Gary's ranch hands, John and Clayton, struggling to get some rivets out of an old hay cutting blade and since they needed another hand, I helped them wrestle the parts off.

Randy Gee, the pilot who had flown me up from Fort Ware, was getting ready to go to the Turnagain Rediscovery camp to pick up the Fort Ware student, and asked if I would like to go along for the ride, an offer I couldn't refuse. We walked down to the gravel airstrip where Randy filled the plane's tanks with gas that he pumped from one of the barrels stacked close by.

Within a short time, the plane was racing down the gravel strip with stones being thrown right and left, rattling beneath us in a most disconcerting way, and then suddenly we could hear only the noise of the engine as we lifted off, leaving behind a cloud of dust that spread out over the hay meadow below us. It was interesting to see that the grassy banks beneath us had eroded, leaving what looked like giant steps all along the hillsides. A deer grazing in some small bushes stared up at us unconcerned and then continued eating again.

The flight to the camp on the Turnagain River took twenty-five minutes through some astoundingly beautiful mountain scenery. In the scree high up on one of the many mountain peaks to the west of Terminus Mountain, we saw trails made over the centuries by the sheep that traversed these precipitous slopes. Three mountain goats clustered together on a rocky outcrop and, on an adjacent mountain, a small herd of Stone's sheep grazed, seeming to ignore the noise of the Cessna.

The Turnagain River was named by Samuel Black when he was exploring the Interior. He had been sent in 1824 by Governor George Simpson of the Hudson's Bay Company to the headwaters of the Finlay River and

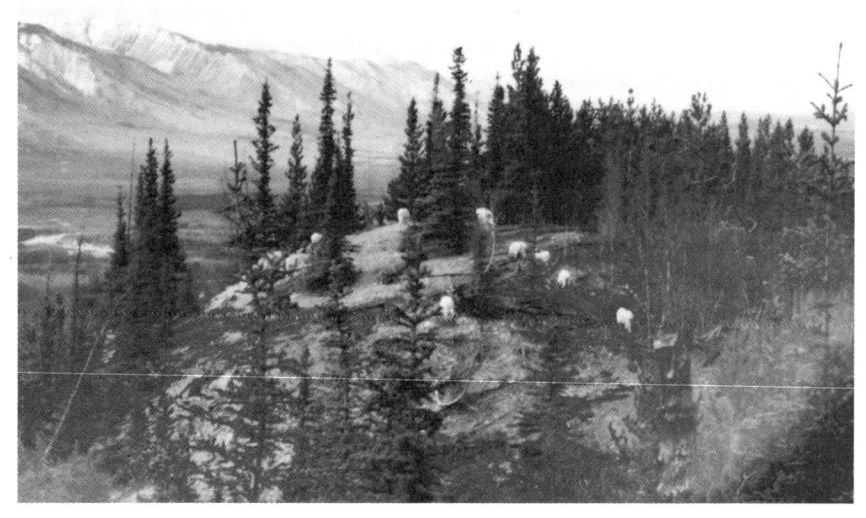

Mountain goats graze on Terminus Mountain.

beyond, to see if the country, in particular the Hudson's Bay Company, could benefit from a new store in the area where furs could be obtained from the local Native people. Samuel Black and his party met an old Chief named Methodiates at the head of the Finlay River at the Fishing Lakes who advised Black to travel north along the Rocky Mountain Trench following the Fox River and then take the long portage to the Kechika—exactly the route that Old Davie used years later. Ignoring this advice, Black travelled past the headwaters of the Finlay, sometimes travelling less than four miles a day. Thutade Lake, at the head of the Finlay River, is incidentally the source of the 3,801-kilometre Mackenzie River.

Samuel Black travelled over to the headwaters of the Stikine River, then over the mountain pass to the east where he came upon a river that flowed northward. Because of his lack of food and his concern for his played-out men, he "turned again," named the river the Turnagain, and retraced his steps to the Finlay. Had he persevered, he would have found that the Turnagain River was a tributary of the Liard River and following it would have afforded him a way to the Mackenzie River and perhaps an easier way back to Fort Vancouver. His journal account of the expedition documents "the extreme hardships faced by the crew and the general privation of the country, both as a source of food and of furs."

We approached the Turnagain River and landed on a very rough, narrow and seemingly too short strip at the Turnagain youth camp and taxied

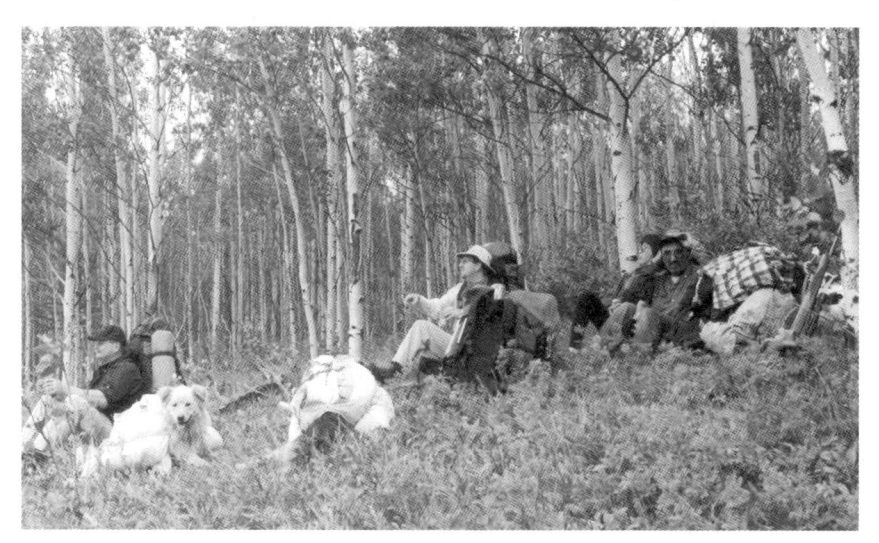

Eric, Jason and Charlie rest with the dogs.

to the small cluster of cabins and tents on the side of the river. Myda Jules, a very friendly Kaska Elder, was busy scraping a moose hide that was stretched out on a large pole frame. She told me that she had been showing the young people how to work with the skin so that eventually it would be a soft, pliable hide that could be turned into moccasins, gloves, or even a jacket.

Myda told us that there were a lot of animal signs around, including moose, black bear and grizzly bear. It seemed a far cry from what Black had recorded as "a scene of tremendous barrenness passing description." He obviously had stayed in the high country and the animals had sought refuge in the sheltered and wide valley of the Rocky Mountain Trench or had migrated to another area.

The student that we had come to pick up was all ready and waiting for us. As soon as her pack was loaded and she was settled comfortably on the small back seat in the plane, Randy had us holding tight to whatever we could find that was solid as we bumped down the strip, the engine racing, the end of the strip getting too close, too fast. I had the feeling that I wanted to make myself lighter so that we could get off the ground more easily, and I willed the small plane up into the air. Randy was in good control and, with some relief on my part, I felt us rise up into the smooth afternoon air. He said that at the end of a warm day the air was thinner and the plane found it harder to gain some lift. Not very comforting information on a warm afternoon take-off on a small bumpy airstrip in the mountains!

On our return to the lodge at Terminus Mountain, Gary invited me to use one of his empty log cabins to sleep in and to go to the main lodge for my meals, another offer that was easy to accept, and one that afforded pleasant company. Joanne, the cook and housekeeper at the lodge, had no other guests to care for that week and cooked a sumptuous supper, after which I went to my small log cabin and tried to sort out what I was going to take with me when we resumed our hike. It was difficult sorting out the food because I didn't know what the others were bringing. When we first started making arrangements, we had agreed that we must keep our packs light and not duplicate things—hard to do when there hasn't been adequate communication.

I packed everything back into my backpack and was rather surprised at how heavy it was. I was hoping Charlie's dogs would relieve me of some things—either that, or I would suggest that we eat the food in my pack first.

Things Old and Things New

Charlie and Hazel arrived by plane at Terminus Mountain the next afternoon and said that Eric and Jason had been delayed with car trouble and would fly up to Terminus later on. They took me down to show me their old cabin on the brink of the Kechika River. The shell of the cabin was still standing, the weathered grey logs standing as a tribute to Charlie and his wife, who had built it all from local materials and without any help.

As we gazed at the old cabin, Hazel told me that a few years ago, she, Charlie and one of their children had come down to the river's edge to look at their old cabin, and perhaps find some willow ptarmigan for supper. Charlie had suddenly remembered that he did not have a rifle with him, so he ran back to the camp to get it, in case there were some rabbits or grouse around. Hazel and her young grandson, Ian, were sitting on a fallen tree waiting for Charlie when she heard a twig break in the bushes and thought that maybe it was a deer. Then she heard a rustling in the dry leaves.

"What's that?" Ian asked.

"Oh, probably just a rabbit," Hazel answered. Feeling a little apprehensive, she told Ian not to worry, there were many small things around in the bush and maybe it was just a squirrel looking for cones. She heard muffled steps and then what she dreaded most came into view just a few metres away.

A big grizzly bear was snuffling around, and coming towards them.

Hazel screamed for Charlie to come quickly. Charlie meanwhile was walking down the trail towards them with his rifle. He heard Hazel screaming something at him, but he couldn't make out what she was saying. He walked a little faster and as his family came into view, he saw Hazel pointing into the bushes.

"Shoot it," she yelled, but Charlie couldn't see anything and thought she must have seen a squirrel in the bushes. As he got closer, a squirrel did run out of the bush and across the trail, but Charlie could not understand why Hazel was so eager for him to shoot it. He had almost reached his family, who were now standing by a big overturned log, when Charlie turned. Still looking up into the trees for the squirrel, seconds later he saw the grizzly bear, now charging directly towards him. He stood stock-still and told me that all he felt was anger at the bear for threatening his family. The bear stopped about four metres away from where Charlie was standing and started to sniff the air, trying to identify this object in front of him.

"No matter what the bear does to me, just stay perfectly still," Charlie told Hazel.

He raised his rifle and then realized that all he was holding was a .22-calibre rifle, which would feel like a pea shooter to a grizzly bear. The bear dropped down on all fours and looked at Charlie.

"Well, here goes!" he said, and Charlie fired the .22 at the bear, hitting him square in the middle of the forehead. To his surprise, the bear shook his head and began running around in circles, thankfully getting farther and farther away from him. Charlie thought that the bear was going to fall over the Kechika riverbank, but instead it turned and hightailed it into the bush. Charlie gathered his family around him and they too hightailed it back to the cabin to get a high-powered rifle, but Charlie never saw that bear again. He told me that the bullet must have only stung the bear, and that the grizzly bear skull is extremely hard. He wasn't even sure why he had fired at the bear because he really knew that it would do no good and could have made the grizzly angry. He was glad that he had not killed the bear, since they didn't need its meat or fat, and he also felt a kinship with grizzly bears because his Kaska family belonged to the Grizzly Bear clan. Afterwards, Charlie went up to the Terminus Lodge and told Gary Moore what had happened to alert him that there was a wounded grizzly bear in the vicinity. Charlie and Gary took their rifles and searched the area without success and then Gary flew over the area with his Super Cub airplane, again without locating the bear.

Some years after building his cabin close to the Kechika River, Charlie had to move it because the fast-flowing water began to wash away the riverbank until his house sat on the very edge. He was worried that the youngest of his growing family would slip and plunge into the muddy waters, where there would be no hope of rescue. The Kechika River—"Tadudze" in Sekani —means "driftwood in water." The huge piles of greying logs that festooned the riverbanks bore witness to the Native name and the inherent danger to anyone who fell into the water. Gary Moore had brought a small Caterpillar tractor into the area, because he wanted to clear some land for a small airstrip. This "Cat" was used to pull the cabin back from the water's edge to a clearing that had been cut out of the surrounding poplar and spruce trees. When they had finished with the machine, Charlie accompanied the Cat driver out to the Alaska Highway, acting as a guide along the narrow bush trail.

Charlie Boya has had years of experience building, renovating, moving and demolishing log cabins, and to my knowledge he built at least eight cabins with very little help. Charlie and Hazel soon had their new house site organized and the trees that had been cleared away from the site were split and stacked, ready for stovewood the next winter.

After many winters of living and trapping at Terminus Mountain, Charlie decided to stay in Fort Ware year-round so his children could go to school and he could be with his growing family. He built himself a log house, not wanting to wait until the federal Indian and Northern Affairs department built him a box-like house. Instead, he designed and built his own, and since there was no community plan to adhere to, he found some land that was dry, with a good gravel base, a source of water close by, and he started cutting and hauling trees for his house. Even though he was home with his family, he said that both he and Hazel still dreamed of their little cabin at Terminus and determined that if it ever became possible they would return to live there.

Charlie and Hazel eventually had a house built by the government where they could enjoy running water and indoor plumbing. Their son Jonathan moved into the old house for some independence and when I started visiting Fort Ware more frequently, Charlie and Jonathan invited me to stay in the old house with Jonathan and they allotted a room to me. This house was in

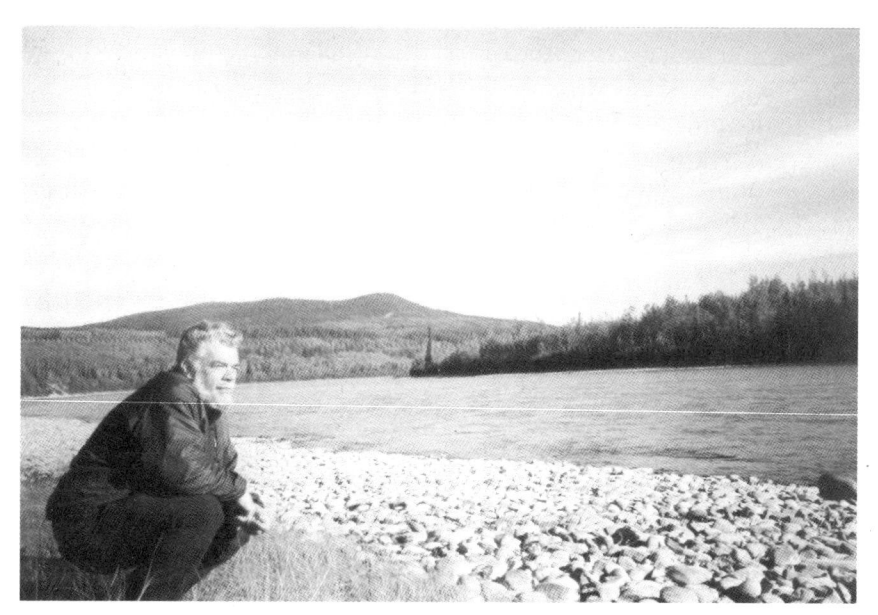

Keith looks out across the Kechika River.

some ways a bit rough, having been built mostly with an axe and a chainsaw. Because Charlie had scrounged or made the building material himself, the house had an authentic old-timer look. Staying in that house was very convenient for me and I knew that I could leave my personal things there without any worries. Visiting contractors often left their vehicles and equipment in Charlie's yard as well, because they knew that no one would touch them.

One contractor parked his backhoe close to the house when he flew to Prince George for a weekend. That was the weekend that the house burned down. Fortunately, there was someone in the village who could drive the contractor's machine and he was able to move it away from the fire before it was scorched. My stuff was not so fortunate but I did not lose anything of value. It wasn't too long before Charlie had a new cabin built on the site, but it didn't have the same character as his old house. There was no official investigation into the cause of the fire since there was no fire department or insurance coverage, but Jonathan thought that it must have been started by the woodstove.

I spent months coordinating plans with the Department of Indian Affairs to provide more housing for people and finally we were able to have a new subdivision built. When the new houses were first built, they were supplied with propane heaters. Homeowners soon found the price of propane too high for their meagre incomes so everyone soon reverted to burning wood to heat their homes and the propane heaters were removed and replaced with wood furnaces. After a huge forest fire killed the majority of trees in the area, the standing fire-killed wood was utilized as a cheap source of fuel and even though so many stoves were being used, Jonathan's was the only house fire that I was aware of in the many years that I was associated with the village. One house did suffer some fire damage after a hot snowmobile was driven into a carport where wood was stored. The wood caught on fire, causing some local damage.

Jason and Eric flew to Terminus Mountain later in the day. They had had trouble with a flat tire on their drive to Fort Ware on the gravel logging road from Mackenzie. The pilot who was to fly them north had to wait for them to arrive, unpack the car and then load the plane—this all caused considerable delay, but they finally arrived at Terminus. They walked with Charlie down to the Boyas' trapping cabin where we were all going to camp, ready to start the hike early the next morning. They hadn't had the opportunity to properly pack their equipment or their food in their backpacks so they laid everything out around the campsite and started from scratch.

Jason and Eric set up the tent they were going to share while Charlie and Hazel set up a mosquito net under a tarp. At Charlie's insistence, I cleared a small space amongst the trapping and hunting supplies in the cabin and laid out my sleeping bag, though I still had my own tent with me and was all ready to camp. Still, I did not want to seem ungrateful for his kind offer. Later, when everyone had settled down for the night, as I lay on my back surveying the cabin's interior and smelling the unique cabin scent of gunny sacks, cooking spices and oil, I thought how fortunate I was to experience a taste of things past while living in the present.

A high wind during the night settled down to a stiff, warm breeze by morning, with a few white fluffy clouds scudding across an otherwise blue sky. After an untraditional breakfast of instant cereal and coffee, Charlie and Hazel carefully fastened canvas packs on the dogs and filled them up with an assortment of food and other supplies while Eric, Jason and I packed up the other equipment. The dogs looked quite nonchalant about the whole thing, walking around seemingly not noticing the added weight in their canvas packs.

Gary Moore came down from the lodge to see us off on this section of our "historic trek," as he termed it, reminding us that it was Friday the thirteenth. We convinced each other that we were not superstitious. Gary had to get back to the lodge and since we were not quite ready to leave, he left his camera for me to take a few photographs. He said to leave the camera in the wood pile and he would pick it up later—one of the advantages of living in the wilderness is that you don't have to worry about leaving things out in the open. After taking a number of photographs, I tucked the camera under a big piece of wood in the wood pile and shouldered my heavy pack, fastened the waistband and chest strap, picked up my gun and set off with Eric and Jason along the trail following Charlie and Hazel. Once again, I felt that I was being pressed into the ground by the weight of my pack, but I also felt excited about continuing in the footsteps of the First Nations Elders.

The overgrown trail from the cabin followed the east side of the Kechika River along a high bank until it joined the Davie Trail about two kilometres farther on. The ground was covered with small prickly wild rose bushes that caught at my legs and scratched my bare arms. Some parts of the trail had been washed out by the encroaching river, so we bushwhacked along game trails, joining the main trail again as it started to climb to higher ground.

Poplar and alder trees grew in profusion, interspersed with a few spruce and pine trees. Deer, elk and moose had scored the bark off many of the poplar trees during the winter when food was scarce and the many pointed stumps showed that the soft fleshy bark had fed the numerous beavers that inhabited the area lower down by the river.

Unlike the country to the north of us, this part of the Davie Trail followed the rivers. At this point, they flowed north, ending up in the Liard River, which flowed to the east and emptied into the Mackenzie River. Later the rivers that we followed flowed south where, via the Finlay River, they would find their way to the Peace River and eventually into the Mackenzie River. Thus, after countless miles, with some rivers flowing north and others flowing first south, then east, then north, all the drainage from the Rocky Mountan Trench would eventually empty into the Beaufort Sea.

We continued to follow the Kechika upstream, its silty water spread out into many channels as it made its way between small islands and gravel bars that had been formed by material washed down from higher elevations. This river had been called the Big Muddy River in the 1940s and is labelled thus on many maps, but no one seems to know when the name was changed, or why. I guessed that the Big Muddy was a name that some white man had given it, and that Kechika was the Kaska name for the river.

Mount Winston, to the west of us, looked almost ominous, very high, with lots of scree below the cliffs. Old snow cornices still clung to the tops of the mountain ridges and one could only imagine the gale force winds that would whip over the mountains in the middle of winter. Most of the mountains that we could see now, and those farther down the Trench, were quite jagged and steep, about two or three thousand metres high on the Trench, or west side. On the backside, the easterly side, these same mountains were quite rounded and easy to climb. Charlie had taken his family to the tops of these when he had been hunting.

After about two kilometres, our trail improved considerably when it joined the main Davie Trail, which ran straight from the lodge. It was well worn by the horses and mules used in the past and now by large game animals. Charlie stopped frequently and dropped his pack with the exclamation that it was hot and we should rest. Hazel whispered to me that it was really because he did not want to tire me out. Comments like this made me feel a lot older than I was, but I appreciated the concern and wondered if some of the early explorers had been looked after to the same extent by their Native guides. I felt that I was in a strange situation most unlike the old days when white explorers hired Native guides. Instead, I was a guest of Native "explorers," who were now documenting their own land.

While we rested on the grassy bank, Goldie, one of the pack dogs, walked rather dejectedly up to us and flopped down by Hazel's side. He was like me, a little older, and needed to adjust to carrying a pack again after sitting at home. Eric and Jason, both a lot younger than me, were quite

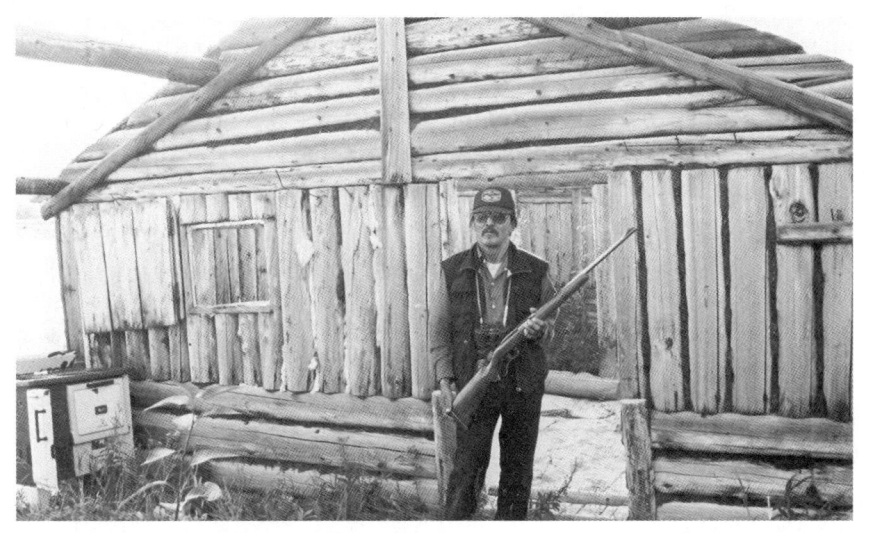

Charlie Boya at his old Kechika River cabin.

happy to stop and rest, and this made me feel a lot better. Eric took the opportunity to record his GPS information on a chart and asked Charlie about various landmarks that we could see.

The weather was warm, with a slight south wind blowing. After a short rest, we continued on our way. A few wispy clouds continued to drift across the blue sky and we were thankful for the continuing good weather. The trail, which followed high ground, was covered with a tough, fibrous bunch grass that was delightful to walk on.

We continued to have frequent rest stops, a fact for which I was thankful as I struggled to get my second wind. Most of the First Nations people that I knew who lived a more traditional lifestyle—that is, they still hauled wood and water and did plenty of wilderness travelling on their traplines or when hunting for meat, instead of becoming couch potatoes like many of their white counterparts—were physically fit and had stamina. Unfortunately, in a lot of areas the traditional lifestyle is no longer in evidence but the resulting obesity is, along with an increasing incidence of diabetes.

We stopped early to make camp. It was only mid-afternoon but Charlie said that the place we had reached was where people always camped, high up on a bank that overlooked a backwater of the Kechika River. This idea of camping in traditional places seems to be widespread amongst northern First Nations travellers. Even though firewood was quite depleted at some campsites, they continued to use them because they were usually close to rivers or creeks and were probably spaced a day's journey apart, as were most trapper's cabins. A few metres away from where we pitched our tents, a small, lively creek took its clear, cold water dancing downhill, where it mingled with the turbid water of the river.

Goldie, the pack dog that had been injured on an earlier trip with Charlie, was slow coming into camp again, and he finally appeared looking quite haggard for a dog, ears drooping, tail down. When his pack was removed, he ate his dog food and immediately curled up under a tree and went to sleep. We had only travelled seven kilometres but I knew how he felt. I wondered if he would be like Jimbo and fail to show up at one of our future camps.

A small amount of meat jerky in a large bowl of noodles, a granola bar, and a chunk of cheese, followed by copious amounts of tea, brought me back to life, so I went for a walk up the hillside, taking Eric's pellet gun along. I was hoping to see some grouse that would provide some fresh meat, but I didn't flush anything out of the low-growing birch that covered the ground, and which made walking difficult, and I had to force my legs through the tight mass of wiry growth. I did find a large elk antler that I brought back to camp, where it proved to be a good conversation piece even though it was quite useless and, as Charlie joked, we didn't really need it for soup just yet!

When I returned to camp, Charlie was showing Jason his skill with a sling and Jason also produced a slingshot. Both of them were pretty good. Our prospects for eating "chicken" looked brighter, if we came across any.

I couldn't help but be impressed by the beauty of the country as we saw the last of the sun's rays cast a red glow on the mountains to the east of us. As we watched the sun's setting rays on the mountainside, we made out two small groups of mountain goats on the grassy slope at the foot of the mountain, their white coats vividly contrasting against the rosy glow of the rocks. They were moving slowly up the slope, stopping to nibble the tufts of grass that grew between the rocks. Our excitement increased when, through binoculars, we saw a large grizzly bear racing up to where the goats were grazing.

The goats did not seem to be bothered by the approaching bear and continued moving, the two groups of goats getting closer together. The grizzly disappeared behind a large outcropping of rock and the goats reached their rocky fortress and safety, although they had not seemed in any particular hurry. Strangely, the grizzly appeared again and he kept racing up the hill past the goats and was soon lost to sight. We could not explain this peculiar behaviour.

The mountaintops gleamed in the setting sun and darkness descended like a curtain being dropped slowly over the scenery as the sun sank in the west. We were left feeling satisfied and looking forward to a night of peace and quiet and then the morning light.

A Grizzly Surprise

The creek was freezing cold first thing in the morning as I washed the sleep out of my eyes. Looking up, I saw clouds gathering overhead. A few drops of rain hit my face, but it didn't seem enough to get things wet, so I ignored it. When I returned to camp, a fire was burning merrily and a large pot of coffee had been made by Charlie, who took Hazel a steaming cup of the brew. Hazel called out to me with a laugh that she didn't get up until after she drank her first cup of coffee. After breakfast, Charlie set off, leading our caravan of hikers. Hazel followed him, the dogs came next, then Jason and myself. Eric carried a new brush cutter that he wanted to try out and he kept swiping at the bushes as we went, so he came last for safety.

The elevation of the land was quite variable because of the small creeks and gullies that led to the river below us. The trail took us through aspen and cottonwood groves where long grasses grew and blue lupines were caught in the tangled undergrowth.

The trail was still easily identifiable as a horse or mule trail. I thought that if it weren't for the blowdown trees, it would have made a spectacular mountain bike trail. We continued on, step after step, and passed below the imposing 2,362-metre Gataga Mountain, its rocky face towering above us.

We stopped and built a small fire in the middle of the gravel trail at Frypan Creek. We didn't want to risk setting any of the surrounding bush on fire but we needed the fire to make our lunch. In a few minutes, we were eating chicken noodle soup and bannock and drinking quantities of plain tea, the most refreshing drink that you can have on the trail. As we sat there around the fire, a few blackflies came to investigate us but maybe we didn't smell ripe enough because they flew away without bothering us, and the few mosquitoes that came were not much of a nuisance. The dry weather helped to lessen the impact of the bugs, and for more than one reason we hoped that it would stay dry, though the gathering clouds looked rather ominous.

The dogs had stayed with us all morning, but after we had crossed over Frypan Creek on a crude bridge made from a couple of logs, we came to an old burn area. There, the dogs soon tired because they had to keep jumping over the blowdown trees. Some of these trees were over forty-five centimetres off the ground, with branches that clawed at the dogs' packs, often knocking the unfortunate animals over. The dogs were not the only ones to have problems. To my dismay, I had a blister develop on my heel in spite of the moleskin bandage that I had put on, and this blight was to stay with me all the way to Fort Ware.

After leaving the burn area, the trail went down a thickly covered track where bearberries and wild rose bushes almost obliterated the trail, but we were glad to see that the tree blazes, though old, were easily distinguished from the natural scars on the tree trunks. A side trail went down towards the river. Charlie told us that this led to a beach where guide and outfitter Frank Cooke used to beach his plane. Charlie and Hazel left their packs and walked down to the river's edge. Eric, Jason and I stayed up on the trail and rested.

After a short rest, we all continued down the trail and I alternated between watching where I placed my feet and looking at the countryside. I took the time to try to get some idea of the places that we passed through, wondering how much it might have changed since Aatse Davie and his family had walked down this very trail. Had he travelled every day as we did or did he stop and hunt every few days? If he shot a moose, then it was likely that he and his entourage would make camp until the meat had been dried and they could pack it more easily.

We could see that the contour of the land changed as we headed for a small canyon and Eric, Jason and I rounded a bend in the trail a few yards behind Charlie and Hazel. Charlie entered the canyon, walking ahead of Hazel, who suggested that they should stop in the shade for a few moments. He had just prepared to sit down when Hazel paused, and without saying a word, pointed forward with her finger....

162   Tse-loh-ne

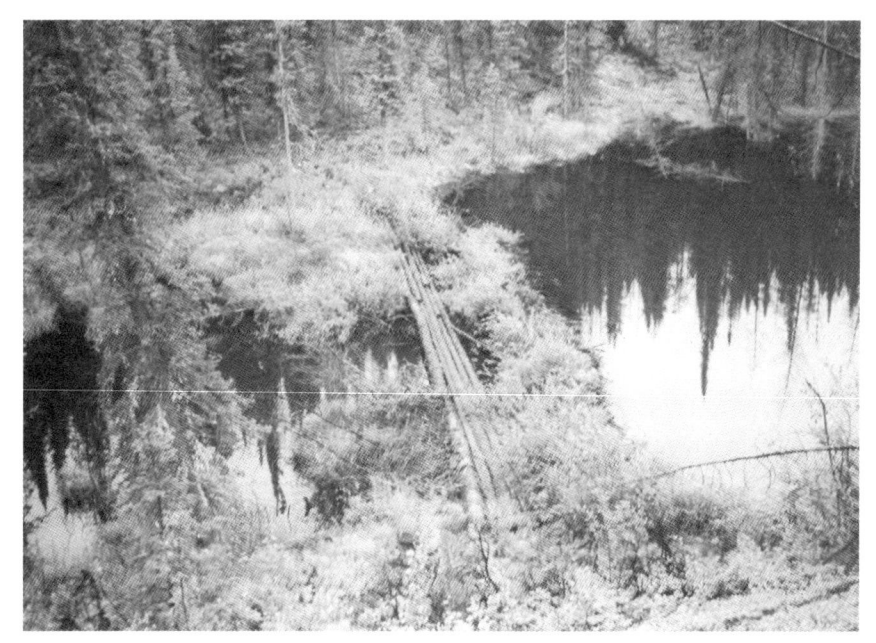

One of the better bridges on the Aatse Davie Trail.

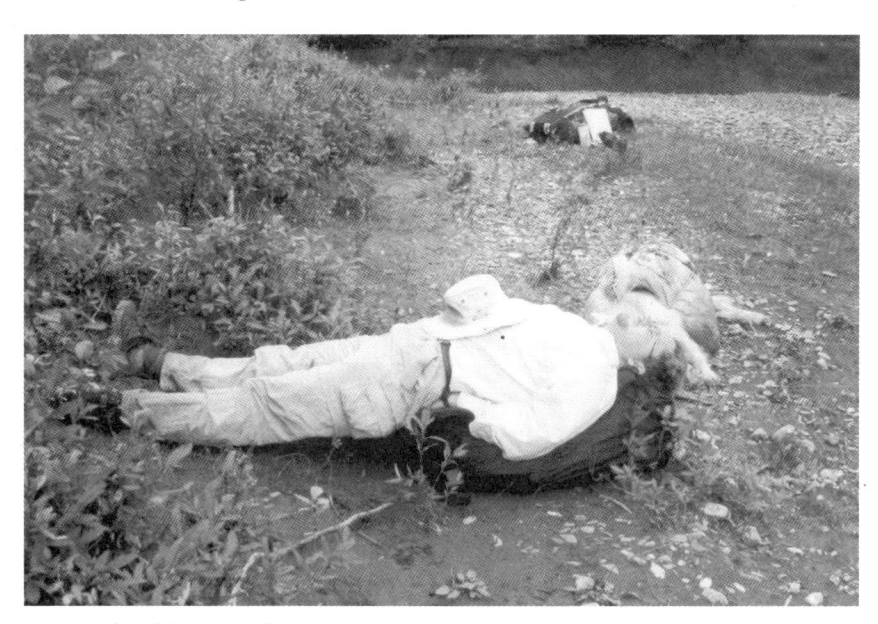

Jason and Goldie pause for a nap.

A large grizzly bear stood up from behind some thick bushes and looked at them, then charged, coming to an abrupt halt a short distance away, then backing up again. As Charlie dropped his pack, he was surprised to see that behind the grizzly bear were two very large, two-year-old cubs, both of them as big as their mother. The sow snapped her teeth, then backed off, only to make a mock charge again. Charlie took the cover off his rifle, knowing that he had only three shells in the chamber. As he watched, time seemed to stand still and he was aware of the sunlight filtering down where it glanced off the grizzlies' golden guard hairs.

"What beautiful animals," Charlie said to Hazel.

Hazel nodded. "Aah," she said quietly.

The big grizzly was now moving slowly towards them, trying to get their scent. Charlie figured that it was time to show this old grizzly who was boss. He raised his rifle carefully, sighted the oncoming bear in the rifle sight, then moved the rifle a fraction to the right, and fired. The bullet hit the ground, shale and dirt spat out into the bear's face, and the loud report from the rifle echoed around the gully. The she-bear stopped in her tracks, shook her head, and turned and crashed through the bush to the side of the canyon, followed closely by her two monstrous cubs.

When it looked as if it were safe, I came up behind Charlie with my two companions. Hazel asked almost nonchalantly, "Did you see those bears? My, they were beautiful!" We examined the tracks, and Charlie told us that the mother must have been a dry sow and that her cubs were at least two, if not three, years old. It was unusual, but not unknown, that they would still be with her at that age.

We all continued on the trail, keeping our eyes and ears open. Even though the bears were long gone, we still felt a bit nervous. Try as I might to not glance back, I had to surreptitiously keep turning around. Charlie and Hazel did not seem at all concerned and I didn't want to look like a wimp!

We came out of the canyon and climbed a ridge from where we could see the Kechika River below us. The ground was covered with low-growing spreading juniper that already had deep blue berries on its branches, a contrast to the bright red berries of the kinnikinnick.

A Grave Concern

As I looked around at the view, I saw what at first sight looked like a medieval sword stuck in the ground just off the trail. On closer investigation, we found that it was the remains of a grave marker. There had once been a low picket fence around the grave. The weather-stained pieces of wood were lying flattened in the undergrowth after years of being covered with several metres of snow during the long winter months, and then buffeted by wind, rain and sun the rest of the year, until they had finally fallen over except for this one piece of wood at the head of the grave. When Swannell was surveying in the area in 1914, he found an identical grave marker near Sifton Pass. That grave was that of a Klondiker, on his way north to make his fortune.

Hazel thought that there had been two graves at this site. Jason excitedly hunted around for clues, but a search for the second grave proved fruitless. After our return home, we heard vaguely that some old-timers knew of the grave, but didn't know who was buried there. In the old days, the dead were usually buried where they died. People on the move with limited resources could not take their deceased loved ones with them, or stay too long in one spot to mourn their dead. The needs of the living took precedence.

There are instances of people in the old days dying close to Fort Ware, and sometimes in the village, they were buried in the bush close by because there was no formal graveyard. Over the years, these graves became neglected and the bush would soon take over the site again. Perhaps because there is more of a sense of community and strong family ties now, when a death occurs in Fort Ware, the whole community grieves together.

There was an elderly couple living in Fort Ware who were hardly ever seen apart. Their caring for one another was apparent to all and the family was close-knit even after the children grew up and had families of their own. I have fond memories of them trundling slowly along the gravel road in the village on their new quad bike. Going to the store or just to visit someone they would drive by slowly, the quad kicking up a fine dust behind them. Then disaster struck. The woman was found to have cancer and within a very short time she had died.

Loneliness is a terrible thing, especially when it is suddenly thrust on you. Joe was lost. He walked around the village, sometimes rode his quad, and he would nod a quiet greeting as he passed, but the smile on his face was not genuine. It was polite. He was grieving for his wife. Within a year he had lost weight in spite of his son and daughter-in-law's care and attention. He was sleeping more and we didn't see him around as much.

I was in my truck one day when a voice came over the radio, saying "Keith, come right away to Joe's house." I drove quickly over and went right in. Family members were gathered in the kitchen and the living room and they made way for me, indicating the main bedroom. Joe lay on his side on the bed, fully clothed. His favourite grandson lay by his side with his arm over him, tears streaming down his face. I felt for a pulse. Nothing. I could tell that Joe was dead but I had been taught to always double-check.

Apparently Joe had gone to lie down in the afternoon. As the day wore on, his grandson became concerned when his grandfather didn't come out of his room and had taken a peek in the room. He had immediately called his mother, who had come over to the house. The old moccasin telegraph and a few truck radio calls soon had people converging on the house.

At this time, the RCMP had a detachment about one hundred kilometres away in Tseh Keh and I called to advise them of Joe's death. There is nothing like a sudden death to get someone's attention and within a very short time, two officers arrived at the house.

"Did anyone touch the body?" one of them asked.

"Of course. Young Johnny here did. Joe was his grandpa," I said, pointing to Joe. Then I added, "I did too. I had to check his pulse and chest." They looked at me questioningly. After all I was just a band manager to

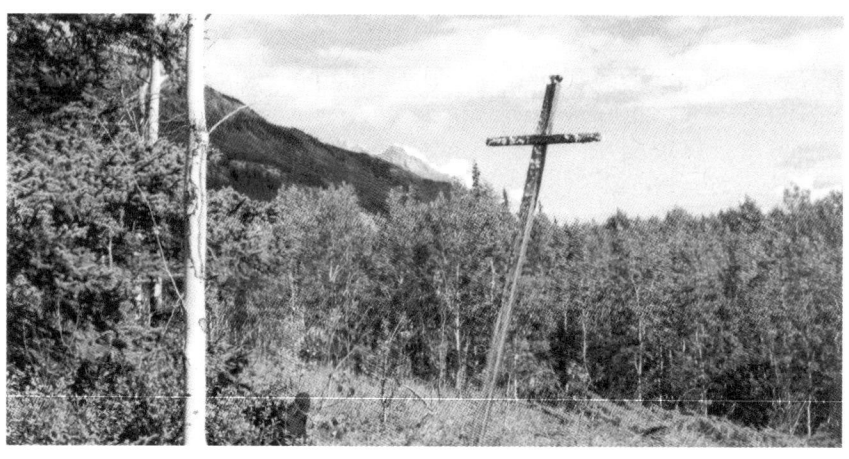

A grave marker rises from the ground like a medieval sword. No one knew who was buried here.

them and they probably wondered who I thought I was, to be examining the body. They took notes and numerous photographs, then finally conceded that everything was in order and left the house.

When people died in Fort Ware they had always been taken to Prince George either for a doctor's examination, a coroner's report or an autopsy, then they would be moved to a funeral home and then flown home to Fort Ware for burial. The costs of this would usually be borne by the coroner's office and when push came to shove, by the Department of Indian Affairs. This time no one would agree to pay to have Joe flown out, placed in a casket and flown back to Fort Ware because there had been no need for an investigation other than the cursory exam done by the police.

"So what are we supposed to do?" I angrily asked the bureaucrat in Vancouver.

"The same as usual," he replied.

I had just told him what had always occurred when someone died so we were already on the merry-go-round.

"Can't you transport the body out on a truck?" he continued. I could envisage an old pickup truck driving the seven hundred-kilometre dusty gravel road to Prince George with Joe's body bouncing around in the back. I hung up the phone in disgust.

The upset family asked me what they had to do, and I told them the response from the government.

"What shall we do then?" someone asked.

"Can you build a coffin out of plywood?" I asked.

"Sure, but what about Joe?"

Inwardly I groaned. I had laid out dozens of people right from the time when I did my basic training in England and then again in Fort McPherson where undertaker facilities did not exist. Now I was faced with a similar situation, and it would not help anyone if I said that it wasn't in my present job description and left the family to solve the problem.

"Get me some new clothes for Joe and I will look after him, but you will have to move him from here."

"How about the church?" There was a small log house that had been converted into a church and where a priest visited the village periodically to hold church services.

Joe was placed on the clinic stretcher and was carried over to the church by some stalwart young men. I closed the curtains on the small windows of the church and told the family to call me when they had the clothes. I went to the clinic and the Community Health Representative gave me free range to collect the supplies I needed.

After washing, shaving and preparing the body, I then set about dressing him in his new clothes. This was a difficult job because rigor mortis had set in and the joints didn't want to bend any more but a bit of constructive (or destructive) work on the clothing was soon accomplished and Joe looked presentable in his new clothes.

A finely-crafted plywood coffin covered with some kind of coloured linen material was brought to the church and I called for Joe's son-in-law to help me place Joe in the coffin. Some white sheeting was fluffed up around him and we balanced the coffin on some chairs ready for people to come and view the body.

Sometimes we had difficulty locating a Roman Catholic priest to fly to Fort Ware to conduct funerals. If we were unable to find a willing priest—which happened several times—John R. McCook, a Band member who was a lay reader in the church, conducted the service as well as a professional. Almost the entire village came out to pay their last respects and many tears were shed. I withdrew so that I would not be caught up in other people's emotions.

People were always very thankful for any help I was able to offer and that made it all worthwhile, though I often wondered how on earth I would write up my job description.

Gataga Forks

After the day's hike of fifteen kilometres and about twenty minutes from the trail gravesite, we arrived at a place that was referred to alternatively as "The Junction," "The Crossing" or "The Forks." The trail ended at the brink of the Kechika River at an old horse corral where the white waters of the Gataga River rushed into the murky Kechika River. The Gataga name was Anglicized from the Sekani "Gah Tahi Gah"—meaning "the river that is amongst the rabbits."

Without losing a step, the dogs immediately waded into the white water of the Gataga, lapping it up noisily, and then just standing in it up to their bellies, panting, and occasionally lapping up some more, probably enjoying the cooling effect of the river water. The packs hung in the water but, as usual, the contents were well wrapped in plastic. As we sank down on the mossy ground, the dogs came out of the river, shook themselves vigorously, nearly falling over as their heavy packs swayed with the shaking, then went and sat in the shade of some spruce trees. After a moment of rest, we removed the packs from the dogs, emptied them and hung the wet packs on the corral fence to dry.

The Gataga River level was higher than usual, and its waters were very silty, rushing down from the glaciers on Mount Roosevelt and Mount Churchill. Washing in the cold water proved to be very refreshing, and some laundered clothes soon joined the dog packs drying on the peeled pole fence.

Tents were erected and a fire started to boil tea water and cook supper. The cold water had been murder on my heels, both of which now had large blisters. The constant irritation from my usually wet footwear, compounded with the weight of my pack, did not give the tissues time to heal.

Between us we had a mixture of footwear. Eric, Jason and I wore hiking boots of varying quality, and Jason suffered as I did from blisters. Then there was Hazel, wearing lace-up Oxford shoes and Charlie with nothing but city loafers—and not a sign of a blister between them. Modern technology has something to learn from this, but I'm not sure what!

Old Davie and his counterparts wore moosehide moccasins and they must have had wet feet most of the time. The moosehide was very supple and very comfortable to wear when it was dry, but after being soaked on the trail, it became stiff when it dried and had to be rubbed vigorously between the hands to soften it again. Of course, all the travel was done on foot so people had tough skin, unlike the pampered feet of us westerners, whose feet are usually encased in hard cow leather.

The crossing was the territorial boundary between the Kaska people of Lower Post and the Sekani of Kwadacha. Louis Boya, Charlie's father, had trapped as far south as this crossing, and Hazel's father, old John McCook, had trapped as far north. It seemed inevitable that Charlie and Hazel would meet each other when they were young, because their parents' traplines met at this isolated river crossing, but it was actually at Skook Davidson's ranch that they first met.

When he was still a young boy, Charlie had moved from the Residential School at Lower Post to the Residential School in Whitehorse, where he completed his formal education. When he was still a teenager, his father had taken him to Skook Davidson's ranch where he was relatively close to his father's trapline. Charlie worked at the ranch for three years as a ranch hand for Skook.

Charlie said that he had heard the name of John McCook and thought he was a white man from somewhere down south. He didn't know that John McCook was a Sekani man, that he had a wife called Minnie, and a young family of three girls and a boy, Nora, Maureen, Hazel and Craig.

When Hazel was seven years old, she and her siblings were taken from Fort Ware to the LeJac Residential School near Fraser Lake. Hazel stayed there for that year, but when the authorities came the following year to take the children away after a summer at home, John McCook (who was Chief at that time) refused to let Hazel go because he said that after one year at the Residential School she "acted differently," adding that "she was not the same little girl that I sent there." John was told that if he would not let her go he wouldn't get any family allowance, to which he replied that he didn't want the family allowance; he had managed before and he could manage now, and he would rather have his daughter at home.

One day John McCook took Minnie and the youngsters up to Skook's ranch for some supplies. They camped down by the Kechika River close to where Charlie's cabin is located now. Charlie was not much older than sixteen or seventeen and Hazel just a few months younger when the two young people fell in love out in the wilderness. A short time later, when Skook could see romance was in the air, he told Hazel, "Honey, don't you go marrying that crazy bastard!" But of course, in time, they did marry and raised their own family. Both maintained a love of the wilderness that to them, even today, is still their home.

I looked out of my tent and imagined what it must have been like to live out here in the old days, compared to our present experience. There would not have been the sound of high flying jets, no chainsaw sounds, or the convenience of satellite phones. There would have been peace, with the wind in the trees and the sound of rushing waters. However, I could appreciate how fortunate we were to live in this century and didn't have to worry about ill health. In an emergency, we could have called for information or a helicopter by using the satellite phone. We had some medical knowledge and first-aid supplies, and we had modern camping gear and clothing, whereas the old-timers had to rely on their own resources and knowledge, equipment was fashioned from what they could find in their environment, and hospitals were so far away that they were as good as non-existent.

As we sat there, Eric pulled out of his pocket a rock he had found close to the trail. The rock looked as though it had been chipped or fashioned into an arrowhead or spear tip, and Jason and Eric discussed the possibility of it being something of cultural significance. No decision was reached. I guess when you have looked at thousands of them, you can tell the difference but I was left wondering if it really was a genuine arrowhead or just another piece of rock.

Hazel told us that when we crossed the Gataga the next day, she would show us where her father and mother had lived and where she had played as a little girl. I looked out over the wide, fast-flowing river, and wondered what it would be like crossing it.

The next day dawned sunny, with no wind to cool us. We worked hard all day but as far as distance was concerned we only gained about half a kilometre. We had hoped that some adventurous people might come by with a jet boat and take us across the swollen river. Charlie said that this was known to happen in some places, and we had seen a boat going down the river when we had wanted to cross the Kechika earlier, but they hadn't seen us and once again we were out of luck. I thought that it was wishful thinking, and couldn't imagine what the chances were of meeting up with someone when we were in the middle of the wilderness and any boat with hunters, fishers or tourists would have had to travel all day in a jet boat to reach here from the Alaska Highway.

The next campsite we were headed for was on the south side of the Gataga River, just below the forks. It was one that saw frequent use (if you can call three or four visits a year frequent), most often by river rafters who paid good money to a commercial outfit to come down the Gataga in a flotilla of rubber rafts. One of the Fort Ware Band members, Hazel's brother, Craig McCook, had been invited to join such a group. Although this was probably for public relations reasons, Craig was a good river man and would have been a valuable team member, both as a guide on the river and then especially when they made camp.

We had thought that with a bit of luck we might meet this group of travellers at the crossing at Gataga Forks, though we were unsure when they were due to start their expedition. As it turned out, the flotilla passed the junction about one week after we had rafted across. Craig later told us that the water had dropped considerably and they saw our raft sitting high and dry on the south shore of the Gataga.

We couldn't sit around in the vain hope that someone would come by, so early the next morning Charlie picked up his axe and I took my axe and small folding camp saw, and we headed up the north shore of the Gataga River with Jason, leaving Hazel making bannock, and Eric catching up on his record-keeping.

Eric had to investigate and then plot an area where a cabin could be built with future tourism in mind. The cabin would have to be close enough to the river for easy access and for getting water, but not close enough to get washed away in the spring flood.

We left our tents standing because we did not know how long it would take to build a raft, and we thought that we might have to stay another night. About two kilometres up the Gataga, we found a number of standing dead cottonwood trees of various sizes, and Charlie thought that we could get enough of the right-sized trees there to build a small raft. When he looked closely at the trees, some had to be rejected because they were either too big or too rotten, but he found a couple that would provide a good start for our raft.

Cutting the trees was no easy task. After Charlie had assessed a tree's potential, a clearing had to be made around it, and then he looked to see if it was leaning in any particular direction. If possible, we wanted to have it fall towards the river so we wouldn't have to haul it too far. Although the wood was quite dry, the cottonwood was much harder to cut than it would have been had it been green. The beauty of these trees is that when dry they were light and floated high in the water. We cut two of the trees down, and then cut them to the prescribed length. Using our axes, we removed the bark and knots from the logs and then, grunting and sweating, we hauled them down to the river's edge. While Jason and I were hauling the logs, helped now by Eric, who had joined us, Charlie cut and shaped two paddles and a long pole that we would use to propel the raft across the current.

The day was hot and the work made us hotter. I was glad we were close to the river so I could frequently drink the silty water. I glanced up the river and was struck by the beauty of the view. The broad river curved around a bend after seeming to flow parallel to the steep mountains. The blue sky served as a backdrop to the craggy mountains and the pine tree-lined river flowing over the rocks towards us was something that is usually only seen on exotic calenders. Following Charlie, we bushwhacked another kilometre or so up the river searching for more suitable cottonwoods, and when we saw a cluster of them, Charlie set us to cutting the trees down and clearing another pathway to the river's edge. The pieces that we hauled out of the bush were nearly five metres long and thirty centimetres in diameter and required an enormous effort to move them to the water's edge.

We dropped the logs into the water and I was rather surprised at how small they now looked bobbing there in the river. Charlie roped them together and then surprised us by pulling from his pocket a handful of large rusty nails. He had come prepared for this. He nailed short poles across the main logs to hold them together and prevent them from sinking when we stepped on one of them. We then had to drift this skinny raft down to where the other two trees had been left on the bank and after we had pulled the two logs into position, Charlie finished tying and then nailing them to the others. Then he declared that all was ready and we went back to dismantle the camp, first sampling some fresh, warm bannock that Hazel had waiting for us. We then carried everything through the bush, the dogs following us happily to where the raft lay waiting.

When we considered that we had four people and three dogs, all of our packs, and needed to leave room to paddle, the raft looked too small and uncomfortably narrow. We knew that we would have to make two crossings. That meant two of us would have to cross the river three times.

Charlie was quite confident about crossing the rushing river on a raft. He had crossed here many times before and had swum horses over. One fall, he had come down to the river on his own and found it running slush ice. Wanting to get across in a hurry (Hazel was in a cabin on the other side) and since the water level was low, he forded the river with the ice pans pushing against his waist.

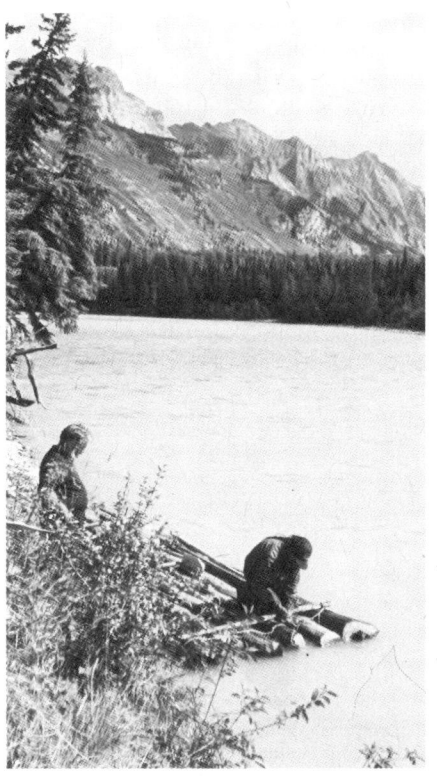

Charlie puts the finishing touches to the raft on which the hikers are to cross the Gataga River, as Keith watches.

He acknowledged that it was a crazy thing to do, but shrugged it off as being one of those things that young people in love do.

Our plan was to paddle up the river as fast as we could until we were out in the middle, then turn the raft around and paddle like mad for the opposite shore and get to the shallows before we were swept into the mainstream of the Kechika, two kilometres downstream. Because the river was running so fast, Charlie decided we would first have to line the raft up the Gataga for another hundred metres to make sure that we could reach the other side before being swept into the Kechika.

I had often read of lining boats up rivers, usually canoes or dugout cottonwood boats, but I had never done it myself. Loading all our packs into the middle of the raft still left enough freeboard, so Jason climbed onto the stern with the pole to push the raft a short way out from the shore, and as the rest of us pulled the raft against the current, his job was to keep it from running into the rocks on the side of the river.

We reached a small eddy where we tied the raft still loaded with our backpacks and the dog packs, then Charlie and I climbed aboard. He went to the "bow" with one of the paddles, and I was given the centre, where I had to sit on the side and provide some strong paddle power on the down-river side of the raft. We grasped the paddles and the pole firmly and agreed that we were as ready as we were ever going to be. Then, with great anticipation, and under Charlie's direction, we cast off into the strong current and from the shore Eric gave the raft a mighty heave to send us on our way.

The Crossing

Paddling and poling like men possessed, we pushed out into the current where we picked up speed—did I say too much speed? I glanced up quickly and, seeing the shore speeding past, I dug my paddle faster and deeper into the swirling river. With every sweep, I hit Jason with the end of my paddle. After apologizing twice, I gave up to save my breath. When I felt as though I couldn't lift the paddle one more time, the raft bumped into a rock about three metres from the shore. Charlie immediately jumped out into waist-high water, and I followed suit, grabbing a rope to haul the lightened raft ashore. Jason stayed on the stern to pole the loaded raft towards dry land.

Once we were in knee-deep water, Jason started to jump off the raft but his foot slipped between two of the cottonwood logs and he became stranded with one foot on the slippery river bottom and the other twisting awkwardly through the raft. We both pulled, but his foot was firmly jammed in between the logs. I bent down and felt for his boot under the water. After finding it, I loosened the boot laces and then he was able to wiggle his foot out of the boot and pull it free from between the two logs. I threw his boot on to the shore to be retrieved later.

We tied the raft to a half-submerged rock and saw that this shore, unlike the opposite shore, had quite muddy banks. It was firm enough to walk on though, so we unloaded everything above the highest water mark, where it was relatively dry. As we unloaded, we were surprised to see hundreds of small frogs, not one of them longer than a couple of centimetres. They were all trying to swim up the river in the shallows, their greenish-grey bodies battling the strong current unsuccessfully.

To get the raft back to our starting point on the opposite shore, we had to line the raft up the river again. Charlie poled while Jason and I pulled the raft from the front. We were all wet up to the waist and we slipped and sloshed over the large wet rocks, but finally Charlie decided we had gone far enough. Now that the raft was going back without a load, it would be easier to paddle, but the current might sweep us down the river a lot faster. Jason pushed us away from the shore and watched as Charlie and I paddled like mad for the far shore where Eric was waiting to help us land. He caught a rope thrown by Charlie, but he had a hard time holding us against the current until we jumped off and hauled the raft to shore, bringing us exactly to the place where we had built the raft. Eric and I pulled and Charlie poled the raft back up the Gataga to the eddy where we were going to start across again with the next load.

The dogs were very reluctant to climb aboard, but obeyed, sitting in the middle looking very apprehensive. Hazel stepped onto the raft and then Eric made sure that everyone was ready before giving the raft another mighty heave with his pole that pushed us out into the current. After paddling in a frenzy again, we headed for the far shore to the same place where Jason now waited for us, wading out into the river to catch the raft as it hit the rocks. We unloaded the raft quickly, the dogs jumping to shore where they ran around investigating the bushes, no doubt relieved to be on land again. We pulled the raft up onto the rocks on the shore as far as we could. Charlie retrieved the nylon rope he had used to tie the logs together and stuffed it into his pack in case it was needed for something else. He left the poles nailed across the logs because he was unable to remove them without a claw hammer.

We were all wet through from our toes to our belts, and our boots and jeans were muddy from where we had hauled our gear away from the river, but since we intended to camp very soon, we did not bother to change our clothes until we had set up camp on a river backwater about a half-hour later.

Travelling down the trail made me realize how arduous the lives of early First Nations people had been. I made the trek for pleasure and found that it made me aware of every sore muscle in my body, but in the end I knew

The Crossing   177

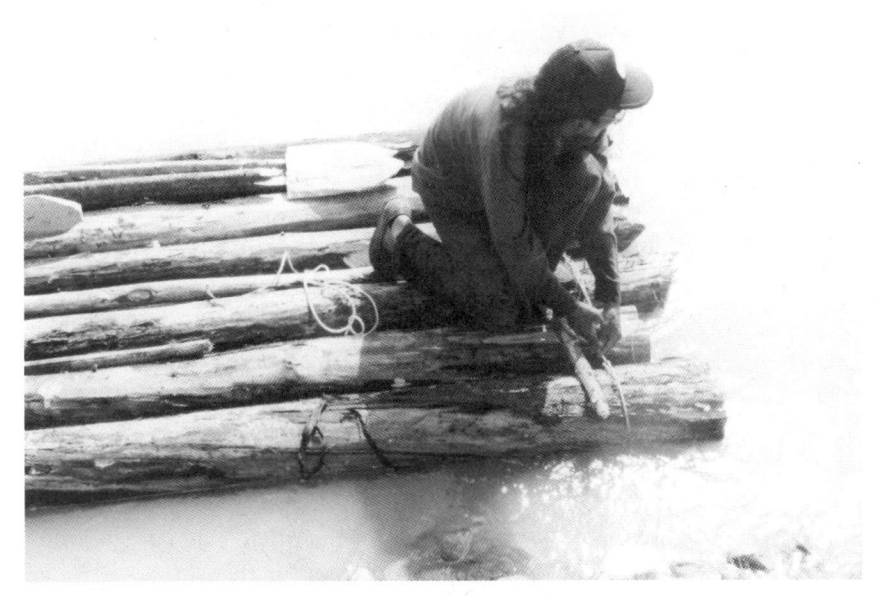

The raft, ready for a river crossing.

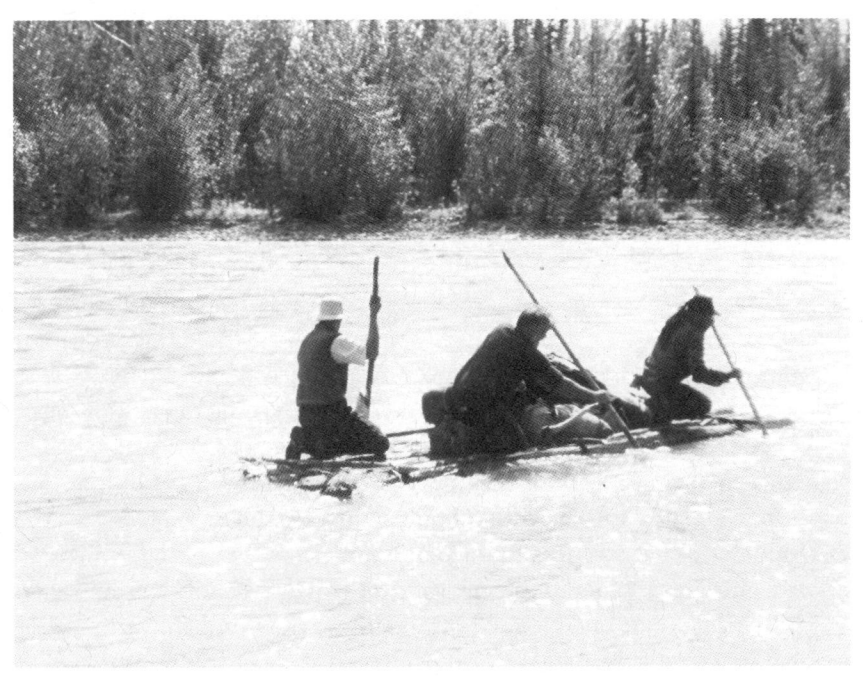

Jason, Keith and Charlie cross the Gataga River on the raft they built.

that I would tell everyone that it had been fun. The people of a bygone age travelled because they had to, not for fun—although they did not travel with the same time restraints as are thrust upon us in this modern age.

Years ago the spruce trees had been thinned out at the campsite, and now soft grass and moss grew between them. Someone had even constructed a "bush toilet" that consisted of a pole nailed between two trees out of sight of the camp. After our camp was made and we had changed out of our wet clothes, I sat on a log at the water's edge and stared at the blue, blue sky and the high thin clouds that floated far above these truly Rocky Mountains, where there were steep rocky cliffs and sheep trails criss-crossing the scree slopes. The forests of spruce and pine nestled up to the mountain base and struggled to reach higher but then petered out when the rocks beat them down. Charlie pointed out two black bears that were cavorting on one of the green slopes far away to the northwest. We stood and watched them for a while through our binoculars, then, when they disappeared into the trees, we turned to contemplate our campfire.

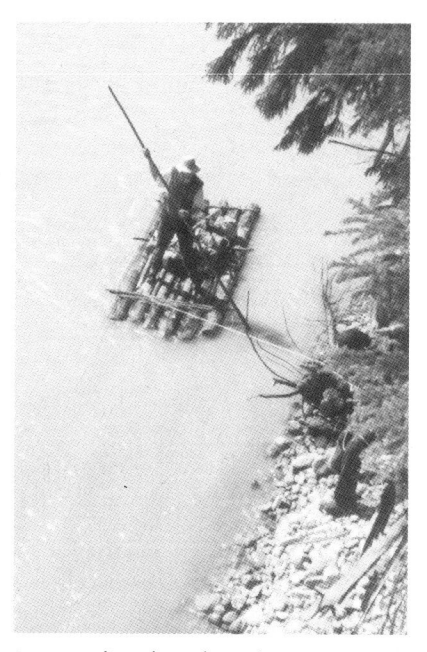

Jason, poling the raft up the Gataga River.

After a meal of our staple diet, chicken noodle soup, bannock, juice and tea, Hazel suggested that we walk down to where the old cabins were and see if her old home was still standing. In spite of my painful heels, I was not going to miss this piece of Davie Trail and Fort Ware history. We had not travelled very far even though it had taken most of the day to accomplish the short distance we had come, and apart from aching shoulders from the hard paddling on the raft, none of us felt too tired to walk a bit farther.

A narrow trail followed the Gataga riverbank for a short way, and then a short cutoff about one kilometre through the trees brought us to a clearing that was rapidly being reclaimed by the forest. There we were at Hazel's girlhood home. I looked at the couple of old cabins almost hidden amongst the trees, and saw that one of them had collapsed.

The cabin that was still standing stood deep in the undergrowth, the old unpeeled logs showing their age, and the thick growth of moss on the roof still able to shed water. A small tree was growing on the roof, nourished by it. One could only wonder whether the logs would rot and cave in first or whether the weight of the growing tree would cause it to collapse. This had been Frank George's cabin—he was a Kaska man from Lower Post who trapped in this area and a friend of Charlie's father, Louis Boya. The floor was dirt and the remains of a small rusty stove stood in one corner, the chimney stovepipes standing at odd angles as they slowly rusted away.

Hazel was disappointed to find that her father's cabin was the one that had collapsed. Years of heavy snow and neglect had taken their toll. Charlie picked up the old door of the cabin, and found the names of visitors faintly decipherable, with times and dates and weather conditions noted. Most of these inscriptions had been written about twenty-seven years earlier.

A piece of tree stump in a small clearing between the cabins had a square hole cut into it close to the top. Although it was now rotting, Hazel explained that it had been where her mother, Minnie McCook, had tanned moose hides. What we were now looking at were the remnants of a moosehide wringer. It had held one end of the large and heavy hide

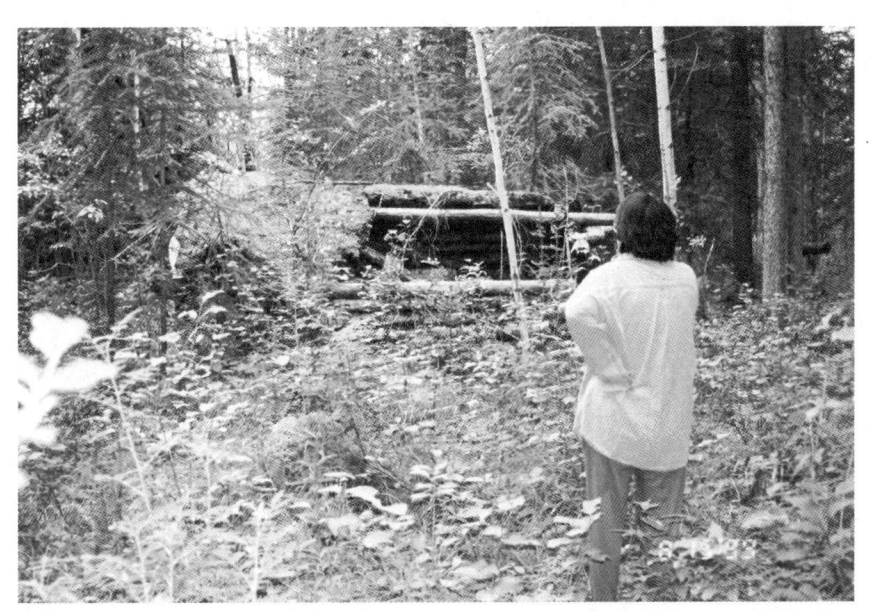

Hazel surveys her father's old cabin, now collapsed.

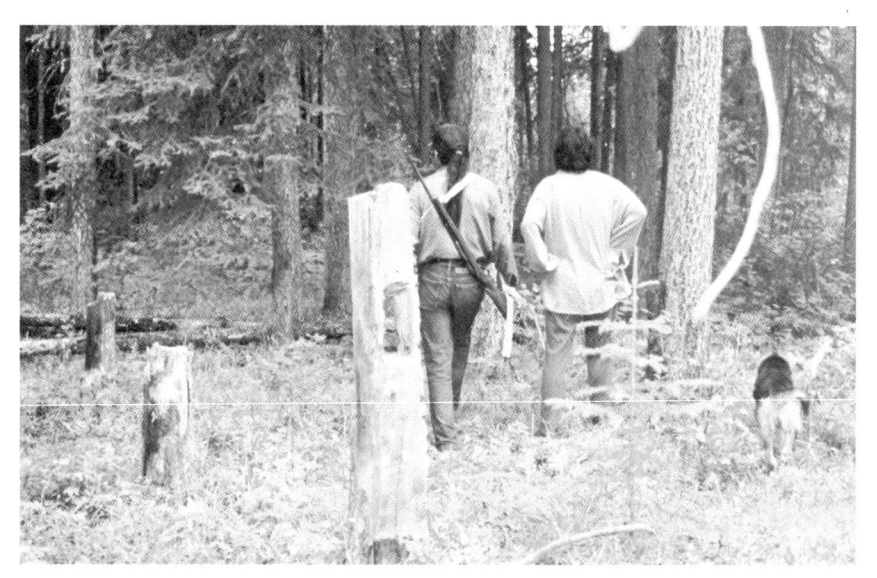

Minnie McCook's moosehide wringer, centre.

after it had been soaked in river water and the hair scraped off, then it was twisted like a pretzel until all the moisture had been squeezed out. When the hide was ready, it was treated with various things—I'd heard of soap being used or animals' brains—then it was spread over a frame of sticks like a miniature teepee, and a smudge fire made inside of this little tent. The result was the distinctive honey-coloured hide with the unique smell that I love. It was then worked by massaging the whole thing until the hide was pliable and soft.

Hazel had spent most of her childhood in cabins like this along the Davie Trail, learning the traditional ways from her parents. How different it would have been for Hazel if she had been forced to go to a Residential School. Charlie and Hazel Boya still rely on what the country has to offer and Hazel especially knew just when to gather berries and herbs. She had been taught well by her mother, Minnie, who was one of the few Elders who used herbs more than any other medicines right up until the time she died at a good old age.

Standing and looking at the old houses, I imagined a young Hazel running around the houses with her brother and sisters, and as usual, I wondered what it had really been like back then. The surrounding trees would have been a lot smaller, or maybe not even there, since most cabins were built in clearings to safeguard them from fire. A number of dogs would

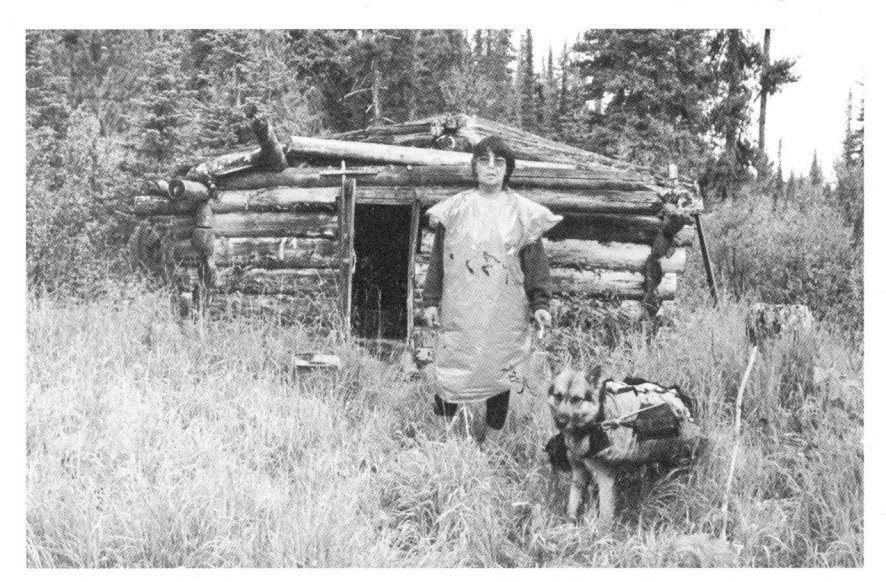

Hazel Boya, in her Fort Ware raincoat, in front of her father's cabin at Sifton Pass.

have been resident here, used as pack dogs in the summer and for pulling sleds in the winter.

I thought again of the horror stories told down south about the Kaska and Sekani people who lived in this rugged part of British Columbia. I suppose that there may have been an element of truth in some of the stories but the storytellers rarely spoke or even knew about the background of these hardy people and the loneliness and privations they endured when they were out in the bush.

City Cabin

After travelling in the bush with Charlie and Hazel, I could see how happy they were out in the wilderness where they used the natural resources respectfully and efficiently. I had been worried about bears and wolves and other unknown dangers, but they took everything in their stride.

We all had many things to occupy our minds as we returned to the camp on the Gataga River and we made the walk back in silence. Our camp was very comfortable and we took some time to clean up and take stock of our supplies. Some food items that we thought were surplus were packaged up and hung in a tree, where they would most probably be eaten by some hungry bear or wolverine. I also left a small but useless heavy frying pan hanging there in a tree.

The campsites along the trail were all different, but they had a few similarities as well. Some had a number of spruce trees surrounding them, others were in predominantly aspen groves. Riverbanks were a favourite place to locate a camp, where there was easy access to water and cooling breezes. Some campsites were just a place to pitch our tents and rest our weary bodies. Charlie always had a goal for us to reach and he wanted to camp where he had always camped. I think this was how he could gauge our progress but it didn't always work out the way he wanted.

At one campsite, I seemed to be dogged by problems. Opening a box of Band-Aids, I found I had only one left, but fortunately I had part of a roll of duct tape that I had put in for emergencies. The zipper on the main compartment of my pack had torn apart when I caught it on a stubborn branch sticking out into the trail. When I had put up my tent and was zipping up the mosquito net in the front door, the zipper fell apart in my hands, having reached the point of no return after many years of use. I took out my repair kit and sewed the net to the tent fabric. Fortunately, there were two doors in the tent. By the time I had finished, the tent was full of no-see-ums and blackflies, and I had to light a bug smoker to clear the tent. Then a contact lens started to bother me, so I threw it away, thankful that I had brought a few disposable lenses with me. I was beginning to see that modern appliances were both a blessing and a curse.

Although we were physically overtired to a degree—at least I was!—we were all feeling some strain from the walk, and still had to adjust to each other's preferences, likes and dislikes. Most of the time we all marched on in silence, each lost in his or her own world. Charlie felt that it was a waste of breath to chatter on about nothing in particular, as most white people do, as though we can't bear the silence. First Nations people on the other hand are generally much quieter. One old Gwich'in man once told me, "No use to talk 'til something to say!" I tried to remember that and to control my tongue, especially when in the company of old-timers. Sometimes I was successful.

I sensed some impatience from Charlie when Eric had to stop to get his GPS readings and then chart them. Eric chose to ignore any untoward remarks and carry on as though nothing happened. He had his responsibility and commitment to the Kaska Tribal Council and a report to furnish for them that would document the Aboriginal right to the land.

We were still following the east side of the Kechika River and the day was good. Too good, in fact, with the sun blazing down on us. All morning we walked out in the open with no trees to shelter us. A few spindly pine trees, small aspens and poplars grew here and there, but nothing provided any real shade. We finally came to a place where large cottonwood trees grew on the side of the river. Many of them had been blown over by the wind or washed out by the spring flooding of the river. We pushed through a muddy section of trail that wound around the big trees.

This was a place that was known as "City Cabin." I asked where the cabins were but was told that they had been built fairly close to the river at the bottom of the hill that we had just climbed, and they had all been washed away by high spring water many years ago. There had been a number of cabins here. By comparison with the isolated trappers' cabins, it really had been a "city," with people coming and going up and down the Trench. In the old days when the Native people lived out on their traplines, there had also been more cabins along the Kechika River, inhabited by people from Fort Ware, and the Davie Trail had been used by people walking, or in the wintertime with their dog sleds, travelling to the village.

Many years ago, one young man, Elmer McCook, had driven a team of dogs, with hardly a break, all the way from City Cabin to Fort Ware, a distance of over one hundred and fifty kilometres. He proudly stated that it was the fastest trip anyone had made. Now there are no more dog teams in Fort Ware so he remains the record-holder. I hoped that his dogs had survived such a gruelling trip. Travelling long distances at a remarkable speed appears to be a cultural phenomenon of the Sekani people from Fort Ware. Whenever anyone returns from walking a trail, the question is inevitably asked: "How long did it take you?" People knew who had travelled the trip fastest and vied to break the record.

Hazel pointed to a long stretch of river far below us, telling us that at one time planes could land there. We looked down at the gravel bars that showed clearly along the river, and realized that it had changed considerably in the last twenty years. She went on to tell us how, when she was a little girl, she and her brother, Craig, would unhitch their dog team when they were coming down the river in winter, and holding up a canvas sheet they would ice-sail down this straight stretch of river.

When Hazel was expecting her first daughter, Carolyn, it was late in the fall. Enough ice had formed on the Kechika, so Charlie arranged for Hazel to fly to City Cabin from Fort Ware in a small plane that also carried their winter supplies. Charlie planned to follow when he could.

Hazel arrived at their cabin and made herself comfortable. Meanwhile Charlie, concerned about leaving Hazel alone for too long when she was pregnant, started walking up the Davie Trail. He walked eighteen or nineteen hours at a stretch, then slept for a few hours by a small fire. He said that when the moon was out and his eyes adjusted, he just kept walking, and didn't even feel tired. He arrived at City Cabin after three days and two nights on the trail.

Hazel told us about one of her other pregnancies and what had occurred when they were living in Fort Ware many years later. At that time, pregnant

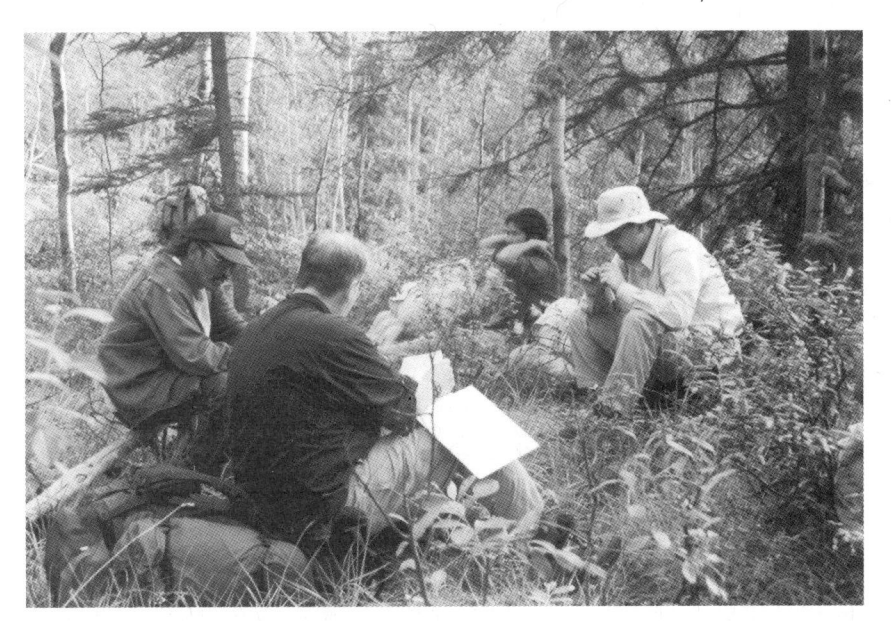

Charlie and Eric discuss the trail. Charlie quietly tolerated Eric's reliance on his GPS.

women were flown out of Fort Ware to Prince George before the birth and most made it before the delivery. For some reason, on this occasion, Hazel was flown to Mackenzie and then told to take the Greyhound bus to Prince George because it was cheaper. Her son Joshua was born on the bus with the help of the driver. Charlie laughed when he added that they should have named Joshua "Greyhound," because now that Josh was a teenager he had long legs and could really move fast!

I could understand why expectant mothers were reluctant to go to Prince George too soon before their baby was due, but so many moms-to-be were unsure of their due dates that the doctor or nurse tried to err on the early side. Some mothers-to-be would wait until the last minute, then if the weather closed in and the plane couldn't make it, the baby would be born in the village.

Not long before we all left on this hike, I received an urgent call to go to the clinic from a concerned Community Health Representative who had been confronted with a young woman in labour. I rushed down to the clinic from the office, where I was working on some Band business. I had time to scrub up, talk to the patient and her husband, and examine her to find out how the baby was faring. Fortunately, everything was happening as it should and the patient delivered a bouncing baby boy, much to the joy of everyone,

Dad also being present for the birth. It was one of the happiest birthing experiences I attended in Fort Ware.

When I was walking along the trail, I often thought about my job and how so many people these days refuse to do something if it isn't in their job description. In the north, it was so easy to do what you had to do and not worry about all the petty workplace problems that seemed to occur in the south. I was quite happy to do whatever the people wanted me to do, especially when there was an obvious need. I know that some people would try to take advantage of my attitude but usually I knew my limits.

Our pack dogs had been on short rations because we had not shot many grouse, so Charlie went off down the trail, taking a pack with him to lighten the load for the following day. He took his rifle and hoped to see a deer that he could share with the dogs. He walked a long way towards the next campsite and came back late at night without having seen anything we could eat. This part of the "Serengeti of the North" was not living up to its reputation and, though we had seen animals in the distance and prints in the mud on the riverbanks, they were making themselves scarce whenever we passed by. I thought of the many times that I had been hiking in other parts of the province and had surprised myself and a deer or two on some isolated trail, but we hadn't even had a glimpse of one since we had left Terminus Mountain.

Boot Hill

The sun was shining brightly on our camp early in the morning and I was up and ready to go before any of the others. Charlie told me to walk ahead on the trail and, besides looking out for bears, to look out for a mark he had made the night before. There we were going to turn off the main trail, which went to a guiding territory cabin at the head of the Gataga River, and the Davie Trail led to a place Charlie and his family had called "Boot Hill." I picked up my gun and, shouldering my pack, set off on an excellent trail, worn down over the years by many feet. I had put new dressings on my heels and they felt reasonably comfortable. I walked along without a worry, not knowing what the day would bring.

I had walked for about an hour and a half and hadn't seen any trail turning off when I heard two shots fired from a rifle a long way away. Knowing that something was wrong and being aware that I seemed to be heading in an easterly direction, I stopped and turned around. I fired my rifle in the air to acknowledge that I had heard the signal. From around a bend in the trail, very close to me, there was another rifle shot that made me jump. I shouted out to be careful since I didn't want to get shot, and then suddenly Jason appeared around the bend. He had heard my shot and thought that maybe I was trying to scare off a bear. He didn't want to walk into a retreating bear so he had pulled out a "bear banger" that I didn't know he carried and fired it.

Jason hadn't heard the first two shots so I told him that perhaps we should wait where we were. He thought that Eric was not too far behind him and since Eric didn't carry a gun we knew that the shots must have been fired by Charlie back at the camp. There were signs of an old campsite where Jason and I stood waiting for Eric. Judging by the horse droppings around the site, we presumed the camp had been made by hunters who had come from an outfitters' fly-in camp up the valley.

We sat and waited, and within five minutes Eric strolled up to us. He said that he thought the trail had veered off just after the last camp. Charlie had put a small tree across the trail, and I could remember stepping over it just as I had stepped over hundreds before. Eric suggested that we could cut cross-country using his GPS but my feeling was that if Charlie came looking for us, he would follow the trail that we were on and would miss us. Reluctantly, Eric agreed. Jason was non-committal. We walked back a long way to where the tree had been placed across the trail. I thought that it really did look as though it had just fallen there. Some small bushes at the side of the trail had been broken, and when we ventured off the main trail, we soon saw fresh blaze marks and broken branches on some aspen bushes.

We followed the faint trail in the dried grass down some steep gullies, jumping over large deadfalls and forcing our way through dense wild rose and red currant bushes, where ground birch tried to trip us up. All the time, we kept our eyes open for the next fresh blaze, of which there were many. It was obvious that Charlie and Hazel were not going to make it easy for us to wander off again. Now that we knew we were on the Davie Trail again, we could see the slight indentation in the ground and realized that we had been too busy enjoying the well-worn trophy hunters' trail to notice this overgrown track.

We started to climb a steep grassy hill, and literally pulled ourselves up using small trees growing alongside the trail as handholds. It was the steepest part of the whole trail and was obviously not part of the original trail that mule teams would have followed. The hill we were climbing had been named Boot Hill by the Boyas. Several years ago the whole family had decided to walk from Fort Ware to Terminus Mountain and even six-year-old Ian Boya, Charlie and Hazel's oldest grandson, had carried his own pack the whole distance.

They had left Fort Ware in the springtime when there was still snow on the ground, and, as they travelled north, taking their time, the snow melted and they changed their winter boots for rubber boots. By the time they got to Boot Hill, the ground was dry and they changed into runners, their rubber boots being all split and worn down. Standing on the brow of the hill, they had each thrown their old boots as far down the hill as they could.

We were all exhausted when we reached the top, so we flopped down and took in the panoramic view while we caught our breath. To the east lay the Gataga valley and the Muskwa ranges, where we had been heading when Charlie had warned us with his rifle fire. To the south we could see the Kechika valley with the Swannell Range and the Omenica Mountains in the direction we were now travelling. To the southwest lay the Big Rabbit River, called Gah-Cho-Ga by the Sekani. To our right, directly west, were the Cassiar Mountains, with the Frog, or Tehkahje Gah, River, flowing from between the Omenicas and the Cassiars to the Kechika River below. Everywhere we looked and as far as the eye could see, the land was covered with green trees, spruce and pine. It was easy to see how anyone who lost the trail could wander about amidst small creeks, large rivers and trees, trees, trees. As we rested, enjoying the view and the southerly breeze, I looked at some bushes behind us and saw where two fresh shell casings had been placed on the ends of some branches. This was the place where Charlie had fired his signal shots.

Eric shot a couple of spruce hens with his BB gun, and he was justifiably proud that he could add fresh meat to the larder. We looked forward to our next meal. As we prepared to continue along the trail, two more rifle shots rang out and I dutifully answered with a single shot, to let Charlie know that we were following. It continued to be a bright, sunny day. Eric, Jason and I were still some distance behind Charlie, Hazel and the dogs. Eric was taking GPS readings, but the trail was good and the weather was pleasant.

Charlie and Hazel had kept well ahead of us, blazing trees and breaking branches from small bushes as they went. As we followed along, we came to a small dried-up lake of whitish mud that, judging by the myriad moose tracks, was a well-used mineral lick. There had been a lack of trees to blaze nearby for Charlie to mark his progress, and now all we saw was this small dry lake. We kept walking ahead, keeping our eyes open for signs of a blaze on the far side. Besides the moose tracks in the white mud, we also saw signs of deer, wolf, grizzly and black bear, but no human prints. We scoured the whole swamp without success and retraced our steps to the last sign. The trail just seemed to fade out completely just before it reached the lake. We went down to the swamp again and I fired three shots in the air, the noise echoing through the hills. No reply.

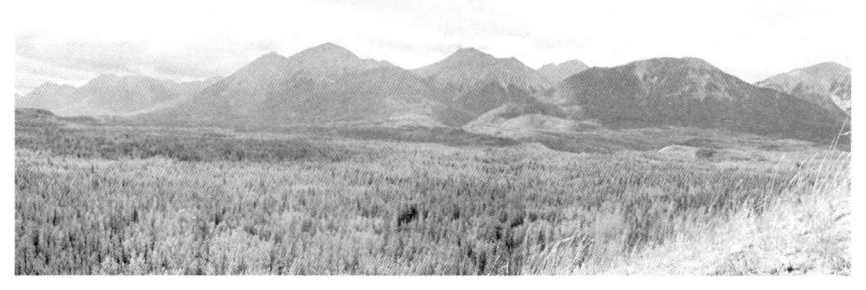

The panoramic view from Boot Hill.

From the maps Eric carried, we knew that the trail had to go southwards with the mountains on one side and the river on the other. So after looking closely at the maps, we bushwhacked in a generally southerly direction, following game trails whenever we could. Coming quite close to the river, along a very high bank, we could make out thick mud and water between the trees far below us where the river had flooded recently. This was not a place where we could get easy access to water, a commodity we all needed desperately at this point.

We saw a very old blaze on a tree and then another, this one quite high up a tree. These blazes led me to believe that they had been made by someone on snowshoes in deep snow. We were on a very old trapline trail. The trapper had to have been going somewhere, so we followed his blazes.

A moose had slid down the cutbank to the river far below, and since we were now really thirsting for a drink of water, we followed suit, slipping and sliding down. After a few metres of fighting through the underbrush at the bottom of the bank, we came to a gravel beach where we sat and rested. I filled my water bottle twice and drank a litre and a half of the cold water. While the others sat on the rocks and rested, I walked up the river a short way to see if there was a way along the shore to the next camp, even though I didn't know where the next camp was. I didn't want to climb back to the top of the cutbank and start fighting the bush again. The river turned sharply just ahead of us and I saw that the cutbank came right down to the water's edge, preventing any passageway. I returned to the others with this gloomy news, and while they were commiserating with me, we heard rifle fire. I wanted to conserve my shells in case we met with an aggressive bear, so Jason fired off one of his "bear bangers," which make as much noise as any 12-gauge shot gun. The blast echoed up and down the riverbanks. We stopped and listened. Only the tinkling of the water could be heard on the rocks.

Climbing back up the bank was difficult, but grasping roots, trees and by digging our fingers into the dirt we were able to gain the top and in spite of the climb we were feeling equally refreshed from the water and from hearing from Charlie again. We continued walking along the top of the cutbank until we saw an area where a rough clearing sloped gently down towards us. I thought that it would be advantageous to walk through it instead of fighting our way through the trees and we were heading for the top of the rise when we heard a shout behind us.

"BANG, BANG, BANG!" Charlie emerged from the trees on the edge of the meadow, laughing and saying, "I could have shot three white men!" He asked if we had heard his shots, which we had. Down by the river, though, we were unable to tell exactly which direction they had come from. He told us how he had broken the branches where he and Hazel had left the game trail. He thought it should have been obvious to a blind man, so we didn't argue, but I thought that we would have to be more observant in the bush if we didn't want to keep getting lost. Charlie told me to give him my pack. I appreciated his help, but couldn't help thinking that Eric and Jason were as tired as I was. However, I was not about to give up one of the advantages of being a senior.

We set off after Charlie with a feeling of relief, walking through cottonwood groves. It was pleasant walking along a grassy trail after the bushwhacking we had just been through and seeing the aspen leaves trembling in the slight breeze was refreshing. It was still hot and the breeze cooled our sweating bodies. I think that I enjoyed it more than the others because I was not carrying a pack—a very pleasant feeling. We reached camp at eight in the evening, feeling all-in after walking fifteen and a half kilometres. We followed Charlie to where Hazel was sitting by a campfire, drinking tea. Charlie set to and cooked us all some fried grouse and Kraft dinner, which we hungrily devoured. I then sat by the campfire drinking copious amounts of tea and resting my aching feet.

Thinking of the distance we still had to go, both Jason and I washed our feet. As we shared the last of the dressings for our blisters, Hazel, who had been lying down in her shelter, came over with a plastic bag full of swamp moss. She said that this moss, which formed long pinkish tendrils, was what her people had used to heal wounds. She told us that babies never used to get diaper rash because this sort of moss was also used as a diaper and invariably prevented infants from getting a sore bum, even when they were sick. She said it would be good for our heels and would help the healing process. We were certainly ready to try it, and made small poultices with the moss that we taped in place with strips of duct tape. It felt cool and quite comfortable, and provided something of a cushion when we donned our footwear again. I had been carrying a pair of runners with me for wearing around camp while my boots were drying, but now I started hiking in my runners and stopped wearing my heavy boots entirely.

While we were doctoring our feet, restless Charlie took his axe and his rifle and, though it was late in the day, he went and cleared some trail ready for the next day. The bush seemed particularly thick and overgrown at this point, and he wanted us to have an easy start. Plus he was always on the lookout for some game. He returned to camp at ten o'clock when it was almost dark.

Lone Creek to Rudolph's Cut Bank

We had walked almost fifty-five kilometres from Terminus Mountain and Eric estimated that we had another one hundred and twenty more to go. Now that's the sort of information that really knocks you back first thing in the morning when you're sitting by the fire enjoying your first drink of coffee and contemplating two great big blisters on your heels. There was no way that I was going to quit and go back. I had wanted to go on this venture and here I was enjoying it, and here I was going to stay! What more could I ask for? Reading about the old way of life was one thing, but to experience it was invaluable.

We soon passed the point that Charlie had reached the night before when he had cut out some of the overgrown trail, then we seemed to spend the rest of the day fighting our way through more bush. I had no idea where we were and most of the time I could see nothing of a trail. Now and again I caught a glimpse of some mountains through the trees, and a sliver of light reflecting on some water, but whether it was a lake or the Kechika River, I couldn't tell. My eyes were more focused on hidden logs and bush backlash—where the person in front lets a springy branch go and it lashes back, whipping you across the face.

I fell, tripping over a large stone, and then fell again, jamming myself into some bushes the second time. Jason, who was now walking behind me, had to lift my pack so I could untangle myself. Jason was twenty-seven years old and having as much difficulty as I was, so I convinced myself that my performance had nothing to do with age.

We came to more cutbanks overlooking the Kechika River and followed them for a while, and then plunged down to the river level before grasping our way to the top again. I think even Charlie lost the trail at one point. He had us rest awhile so that he could go and locate it again, or cut a rough new one for us.

I got quite used to the way Charlie would sometimes stop for a moment, look around in front of him, and then push his way through what seemed like impenetrable bush until all I could see through the trees was his huge pack supported by his two legs. After realizing that it was possible to force your way through even the thickest-looking bush if you were determined enough, I followed Charlie's example and got quite adept at the technique.

In the mid-1990s, two young men from the United States set out to walk down the Davie Trail from Terminus Mountain to Fort Ware. In a letter they sent to Charlie, they wrote: "The trail eventually led us to a boggy swampy area and as we went deeper and deeper into the swamp the trail seemed to fade and we began to follow one ghost trail after another. It is difficult to explain in vivid enough detail the event(s) of the next two days, hell comes to mind as does torture." Only when they met Charlie at Fox Lake did they learn that they had been following the winter dog team and snowmobile trails that most of the time crossed frozen swamps and followed creeks and rivers.

It started to rain after lunch and we donned our rain gear, which, as usual, didn't do us very much good because we were just as wet from sweating. When the shower had passed, I took off my wet things and slipped them into the straps of my pack. Again I thought of the old-timers who didn't have the waterproof clothing that is available today and who wore deer or moosehide clothing that would be difficult to dry. In spite of the wet and discomfort, I was glad to be travelling today.

We reached Lone Creek by mid-afternoon after hiking about twelve kilometres. Although I don't think it was Charlie's preferred campsite, I was quite happy to stop there. Charlie found enough room on the riverbank for us to set up our shelters amongst the trees where the moss was knee-high. Once a few branches and twigs were cleared away, we had wonderfully soft mattresses.

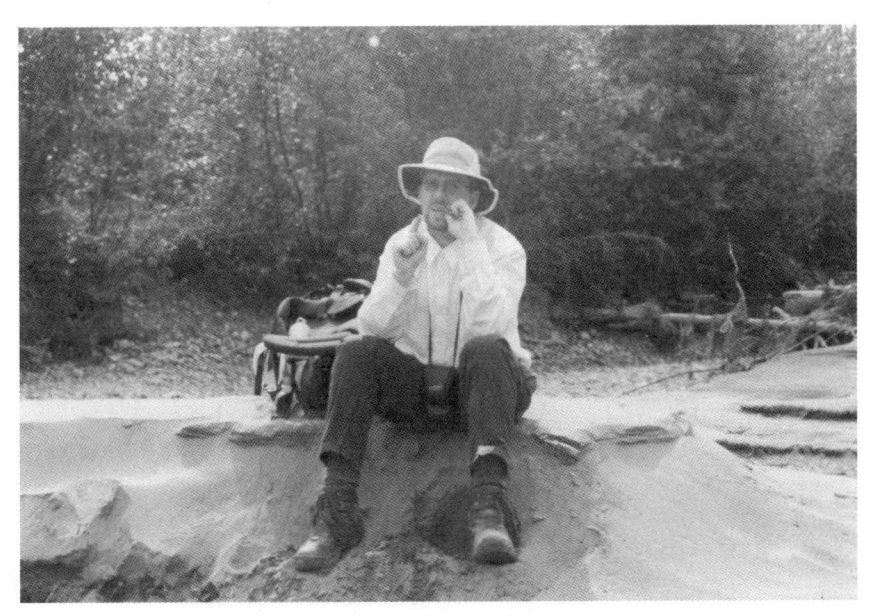

Jason plays a tune on his "Jew's harp."

I asked Hazel where Lone Creek really was because we hadn't passed a creek in this vicinity, and I couldn't hear any rushing water other than a bit of noise from the Kechika. She told me that Lone Creek was really on the other side of the river. They called this Lone Creek because her dad, John McCook, called the large mountain to the west Lone Mountain, because it stood very much alone.

We were sitting down on the riverbank when I heard a peculiar twanging noise coming from where Jason was sitting. Intrigued, I went over and found him playing a small mouth instrument that he said was a "Jew's harp." It was the sort of sound that would have gone well with a homemade bass, constructed with a box, a broom handle and length of twine, but those items were a long way off. Entertainment out in the bush was whatever you made it!

We had been discussing the number of bear tracks we had seen in the area. Afterwards, Charlie came and fastened Bruno close to my tent, and I felt that Charlie and Hazel were making sure that I was safe. I was grateful for their concern and care. Hazel told me later that when we had been lost the day before, Charlie was worried about me and came to help. He thought I was going to have a heart attack with the strain, and then he would have felt responsible for inviting me along.

I had just finished doing my laundry and hanging it up to dry when a dark cloud cast its shadow over us and it began to rain heavily. It rained all night and the clothes I had washed were now so wet I had to wring them out and pack them in a plastic bag. They were now a lot heavier too. Anticipating that it would rain, I had hung some underwear in the tent when I went to bed, then when I awoke, I put the very damp clothes on my chest to help dry them. After all, that's what the books say to do. When I got dressed a half-hour later, I was able to put on warm, damp underwear.

If I thought that the day before had been tiring and rough, Hazel advised us at breakfast time that the trail between Lone Creek and Sheep Creek was the worst part of the Davie Trail because beaver were constantly flooding the area. The water usually came right up to the base of a high bluff that we would have to climb and large downed cottonwoods would make our passage very difficult.

We spent the day bushwhacking. Even when we came to some semblance of the old trail, we were knee-deep in moss and constantly had to heave ourselves and the dogs over or around fallen trees. Sometimes the trees were so close together that it was difficult to manoeuvre through them with a pack on. As I squeezed between two very stubborn, unbendable trees, I could not help but think that if the land claims are to depend on the premise of frequent use of the land, then this particular section did not reflect it.

With some relief, we were able to walk for a few minutes along the side of the river. Numerous moose and wolf footprints dotted the sandbars and I saw one grizzly bear paw indentation in the soft mud that was one and a half times broader than my hand span of twenty-three centimetres. The bear's paws had sunk deeper into the sand and mud than my feet had, and I was carrying a heavy pack—giving an indication of the weight of the beast. I was quite happy just to view his tracks.

The sight of the bear tracks on the side of the river prompted Charlie and Hazel to tell us some stories about their bear encounters. Close to where we stopped for a lunch break, John McCook had once stopped for a break with his young family. Nora Massettoe, Hazel's sister, had run up the steep bank only to be met by an unsuspecting grizzly bear running down that same hill. The bear ran off and Nora ran crying to her mother.

On the trip that the Boya family had taken from Fort Ware to Terminus Mountain, they had all been sitting on the side of the river having tea when a big grizzly came out of the bush on the other side of the river, splashed into the water, and swam across right towards them. Seeing it coming, the usually boisterous six-year-old Ian Boya threw a coat over his head. The grizzly came ashore, shook himself and then stood upright, as it tried to get their scent. Sensing danger, it then took off at high speed, crashing through the dense brush. Hazel said Ian stayed quiet for a day and a half after that.

We reached Grizzly Creek where we had to ford the narrow, fast-flowing but shallow creek. Charlie surprised us when he said he had come prepared and had some Fort Ware hip waders with him. Then we all burst out laughing when he showed us two green garbage bags that he pulled on over his boots and legs. He splashed through the water and took them off on the other side of the creek, showing us that he was quite dry. He put a stone in each of the bags and threw them over for Jason to try. After Jason had crossed the creek, he threw the bags over for me. I put them on and waded through the water and felt the water soak through my runners. One plastic bag had torn on a rock and let the water in, but I wasn't as wet as I would have otherwise been. Eric took off his boots and waded across, the rocks digging into his feet, and when he reached the other side he told us the water had been painfully cold.

We sat by the creek and waited for Charlie to scout the trail. I thought it was quite uncanny how he could walk through the bush with his huge pack and rifle and find clearings and game trails, all without a compass. Then I remembered that he had travelled along this part of the trail many times before, and though it was not clearly marked or had been flooded out by the industrious beaver, Charlie knew in a general sense which direction to take by the various features of the land.

I was beginning to flag by late afternoon and mentioned to Hazel that I was worn out. Eric and Jason had trudged doggedly on without complaint and I envied them their stamina. A few minutes later, Charlie asked Hazel if she was tired. She answered that she wasn't too bad, but that "Keith couldn't go much further." I felt a bit embarrassed by her confession on my behalf, but it was true, even though we had only travelled ten kilometres that day. Charlie had hoped to get as far as Sheep Creek but when we came to a bluff that was going to take some roping up to get by, Charlie sang out, "Camp time!"—music to my ears. As we were setting our tents, the late afternoon sun began to shine, so I put up a line and dried most of my clothes.

You can learn a lot about yourself on an expedition like this trek down the Davie Trail. I thought of the times when one or the other of us (I was embarrassed to think that it was mostly me) had seemed a bit selfish, or had wanted to be left alone, or seemed to choose the nicest piece of meat,

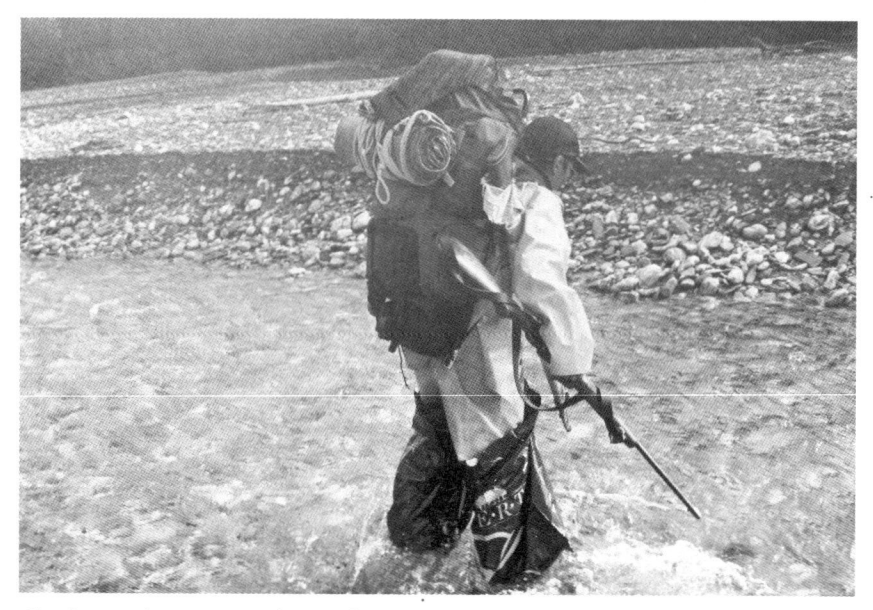

Charlie puts his Fort Ware hip waders to use as he crosses Grizzly Creek.

or looked at the campsites and wondered which place would be the most comfortable, or maybe the safest. I know I did all of these at least some of the time. There was no need for these thoughts though, because, really, we shared everything and I was more than well cared for by the Boyas. Human nature is difficult to overcome sometimes! With these thoughts coursing through my mind, I looked out of my tent door at the river rushing by a few metres away. When I looked up, I could see the sun playing in the leaves of the overhanging branches. The dogs were resting quietly on their mossy beds like the rest of us. I guess I dozed off.

Waking up from my catnap, I heard the sound of chopping coming from the bluff that we had to get around in the morning. I wandered over to find Charlie cutting a way through the brush to the bluff. As I watched, he fastened some poles to make handrails and strung a rope across the base of the bluff. He said that if we were careful we would find enough footing to get across if we hung on to the rope. We walked back to camp and sat with the others around the campfire until it was almost dark.

The next morning, after a good night's sleep, an adequate breakfast and, more importantly, a dry, sunny day, we carried everything over to the side of the bluff where Charlie had tried to make a safe passage for us. He made several trips carrying the dog packs, then he carried my pack over, saying that

I was heavy and might slip on the shale. Sometimes the truth strikes home, but I had to laugh. Jason shouldered his pack and then, followed by Eric, they climbed carefully over the slippery trail making full use of Charlie's safety rope. The dogs were let loose and made their way over without any difficulty and then stood waiting to have their packs put on.

We were not quite halfway from Terminus Mountain to Fort Ware. According to Eric's GPS, we had travelled eighty-six kilometres and had another eighty-nine to go. The last few days had given us some pleasant weather, but it seemed that on most of this trip I was either wet with sweat or wet with rain. When it did rain, I wore my rain gear with the arm vents open but even so I soon perspired heavily and all my clothes got wet. Whenever I had been out in the bush for a long time, I found that my clothes got a little ripe with wood smoke and perspiration. This was not too noticeable out in the bush but became very obvious after arriving home and piling up the clothes in the laundry room, ready for washing. Ah, the beauties of outdoor living!

We followed Charlie and Hazel on a good trail all morning, a trail animals had used with some frequency, until we came to a small rushing creek with thick willow bushes on either side of it. Erik, Jason and I stopped to fill our water bottles and I did not take any notice of the direction that Charlie and Hazel took, assuming that the trail went straight ahead. Then, when we were ready to leave the creek, I saw that there were at least four trails to choose from. The animals that had come to the creek to drink had gone off in different directions, leaving identically worn trails.

Getting lost was getting to be a bit tedious. I thought the best thing to do was to follow the trail that seemed to lead straight on, because it was only rarely that human trails took a very sharp turn after coming to something like a creek. Even in open areas of meadow where there were no trees to mark a trail, I would walk directly across, and usually came out within a metre or two of the blazed trail. However, as we had experienced before at the dry lake, there were times when logic failed.

The trail signs slowly disappeared as we got farther into the bush. Eric thought that we should head southeast and that I was heading too far to the west. Even Jason felt that I was going in the wrong direction, but I felt that Charlie would be on a trail closest to the river and the river would not lead uphill to the east. I didn't want to trust the GPS readings even if Eric could get satellite contact from where we were in the trees, because I had never used a GPS and I was a bit biased. I wondered if Charlie went ahead sometimes to make a point about knowledge of the country versus the technical instruments of the white man.

When in doubt, fire! So before Charlie got too far away, I fired my rifle to get some indication from him which direction we should take. I heard an answering shot from the southwest and we all trooped off in that direction, my bush instinct having been vindicated for once.

There had been some talk of camping at Sheep Creek, but we were unsure whether we had passed it or not. We should have passed a place called Smokehouse first, but, like most of the traditional places, there was nothing to indicate where it was. Charlie was sure we had already passed the creek. Looking at the map and then the surrounding countryside, I couldn't tell one mountain from another and numerous creeks were shown on the map. The confusion was cleared up later when it was explained that Sheep Creek—named by John McCook because every fall the sheep came down there—was called Braid Creek on the map. A better scale map would not have been more useful because the creek's name would have been the same. As it was, I didn't care whether we had passed it or whether it was still in front of us because as long as we followed the trail, we would eventually reach our next campsite.

We came down to the Kechika River again and the trail wound around the trees on the very edge of the water. Goldie fell in while trying to get a drink but we fished him out quickly. We hardly had any food left by this time so there was not very much that could get wet. There was supposed to be a food cache waiting for us at Burn Cabin, where we hoped to replenish our supplies.

I was not aware of passing another creek so I had to assume that Sheep Creek was indeed behind us. That evening we made camp after travelling twelve kilometres. The site was on a dry, flat, grass-covered bank next to a part of the Kechika that was shallow and just invited us to take a bath.

The name of this place was Rudolph's Cut Bank. Behind us a steep cutbank stood out against the sunny sky. At first I could not find out who Rudolph was. Charlie and Hazel agreed that as far as they knew, it had always been called that. Later, another old-timer friend, Tommy Poole, said he thought it was named after some white man. For it to have been so called, there must have been a story there. This name gnawed at me for some time. Years later, after searching around and asking questions, I found that it was named after a Rudolph Forsberg from Lower Post who had apparently been shot there under some questionable circumstances that were never solved satisfactorily. There is a Forsberg Ridge and a Forsberg Creek in the vicinity but whether they were all interrelated is not known.

After eating a rather meagre meal, Eric and I went down to the river and had a good wash. While we were at it, we washed our clothes too. As we toiled away, we heard some trees falling and what sounded like boulders being rolled into the creek. Thinking that it must be Charlie cutting wood or making trail, Eric called out to Hazel in her camp to see if she knew where Charlie was. To our surprise, it was Charlie who answered.

He came out of his shelter carrying his gun, having also heard the commotion down by the creek, and walked down to where I was still standing in the water. He then walked slowly up the river to the sound of more trees and rocks being thrown around. In my imagination, I could see a big, hungry grizzly bear tearing the riverbank apart looking for tasty roots, or maybe searching for some animal hiding in a log jam.

A huge crash came from farther up the river and Charlie came running back towards us, calling for me to get my rifle. He thought it might be a grizzly bear pushing over a rotten tree, looking for ants. I ran and grabbed my rifle, putting a shell in the breech. We sat and listened. Nothing. We both kept our rifles handy, but after fifteen minutes without any noise we unloaded, but kept the guns close at hand. I hurriedly put some more clothes on in case the bear appeared and we had to run!

That evening Charlie took his rifle and walked along the river a short way, then came back and said that he had seen some big black bear prints in the mud, lots of fresh beaver cuttings and newly felled trees. We wanted to believe that the noise had been made by the beaver felling trees onto the rocky beach. It sounded the most logical explanation, although I did wonder about the rocks rolling. I slept that night with my ears on full alert and my rifle by my side.

In the morning I awoke to the sound of heavy rain beating down on my tent. I looked out and the first thing I saw was my line of washing hanging there. It wasn't just dripping, the water was pouring off in rivulets, and spattering on the ground.

I did not want to get up.

Helicopter Evacuation

It rained all day. The foliage was wet, the trees dripped, and water poured out of the leaves when you touched them. The moss was like a soaking wet sponge, and the tiniest creek was transformed into a mini-torrent.

We left camp early, after packing wet clothes, wet tent, and wet everything into our packs, which were soon equally wet. We walked through dense brush on the side of the Kechika River and then squeezed by a slippery landslide, the trail crossing boulders that lay precariously stacked on what was left of the riverbank. Charlie kept checking on us in case we fell into the water, but the water looked less than a metre deep and we couldn't have gotten any wetter than we were already. Now and again, through the rain and the trees, we caught sight of the misty outline of mountains and some high, sandy bluffs to the west.

To compound our misery, many trees had fallen across the trail on this stretch, and were hung up at various heights. I had to walk like an Olympic hurdler, with my leg almost lifting at a right angle to get over some fallen trees. I could feel the wet fabric of my pants resisting when I tried to lift my leg over a particularly high hurdle.

The dogs faithfully followed us until an obstacle was beyond their ability to jump it, or too low to duck underneath it. Then they would just wait until we helped them over. The rain and the wet bush did not seem to bother the dogs at all. When they stopped, they shook their wet coats vigorously, making their packs bounce around, and they would lick their feet. When it was time to move off again, they would wag their tails in anticipation of another stroll.

We came to a swollen creek called Big Creek, which it certainly was, and Charlie removed the dogs' packs. Following Charlie's example and using poles to brace ourselves against the current, we carried the packs over, then the dogs jumped in and swam after us. We waded back across to get our own packs, still wearing our footwear and socks which didn't seem to get any wetter. When we had collected everything together, the dogs were repacked and we started walking again at a brisk pace to keep ourselves warm. It surprised me that once they had swum the creek, the dogs shook themselves and then walked around us wagging their tails as though they were having the time of their lives. They then stood quite still as Charlie and Hazel fastened their very wet packs on again.

Whenever things seemed to be tough, my mind invariably went back to the old-timers who would have suffered the same heavy rains and miserable conditions as we were experiencing now, and without the modern equipment and clothing that we have. What would they have used instead of a lightweight tarpaulin? Or easily erected nylon tents with bug screens and waterproof fly sheets? Were the "good old days" really good, or was this a romantic notion formed by the generations that followed them?

We came to a stop under the shelter of some big evergreens. While we took advantage of the respite from the rain, Charlie fastened a tarpaulin under some trees that made for a better shelter. Then he lit a huge fire so that we could dry off a little. The tarp had the added benefit of reflecting some of the heat from the fire back down to us. We still had a few packages of soup and it wasn't long before we were drinking a scalding hot meal. Hazel said that perhaps she had enough ingredients to make some bannock when we camped for the night, a good incentive for us to keep going. Leaving the heat of the fire was difficult to do because we then felt colder than we had before.

Still walking through a heavy drizzle towards Burn Cabin, I suddenly recognized the part of the trail that I was walking down. It was like an epiphany. One minute I was slogging through unrecognizable bush which all had a sameness to it, then walking around a tree, I saw a blaze near a peculiarly shaped willow bush and suddenly I knew where I was. It was like being dropped into a familiar neighbourhood.

The previous winter I had been snowshoeing with a friend, Donald Gordon. We were travelling north from Burn Cabin where we had been camping after snowmobiling from Fort Ware and this was the place where we had turned around to go back to the camp. Now it was quite comforting to see something that I recognized, because I knew for sure that we would be at our next camp within the hour.

Just when my spirits had risen, Jason stumbled over a log and twisted his ankle badly. He didn't want to stop, and hobbled painfully the next few kilometres to Burn Cabin ("Koh Wuk'edaludi" or "burned cabin"). We had managed fourteen kilometres when we all literally staggered into camp.

Burn Cabin was a misnomer. It had been built in an area that had been burned in a forest fire, and the trees used to build the cabin walls were fire-blackened though the cabin itself had never burned. There was no roof—it had never had one—and the floor was dirt. The walls were only a metre and a half high, the "cabin" only about twelve metres square. It was built on what had been the brink of the Kechika River, but the river course had changed during one of the many high, fast spring runoffs and was now over ninety metres away from the cabin. A swamp lay at the foot of the bank.

About thirty years previously, Charlie had been asked to build a small airstrip at this site. He and another man had worked hard clearing enough land to the north for a Piper Cub to land on. As they cleared the land,

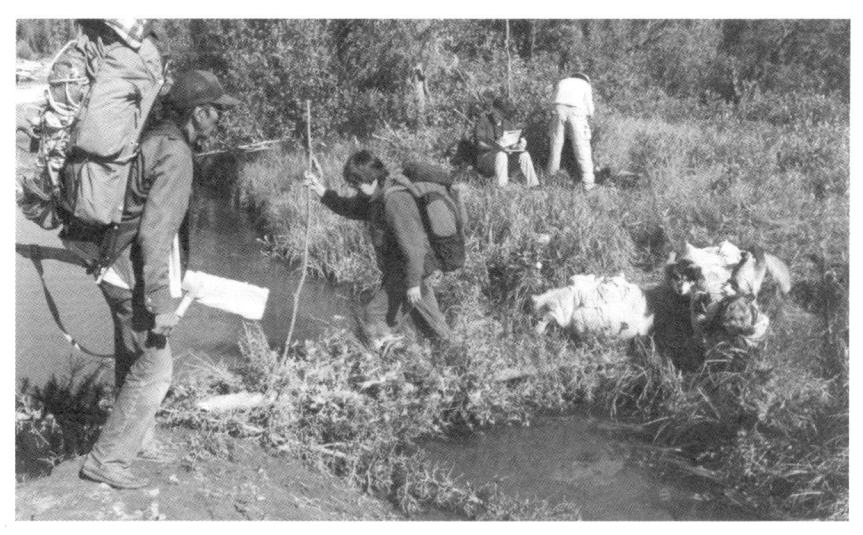

Hazel crosses the creek, steadying herself with a walking stick as Charlie watches.

they found a small narrow creek running across the middle of the proposed airstrip. The creek meant that it would be impossible for a plane to land and equally impossible for heavy equipment to get there to level the strip. Nature was beginning to take over this area again and the bush now reached four or five metres high in places so we knew that no fixed-wing aircraft would ever be able to land there, even in an emergency.

While I looked at Jason's foot and applied a tensor bandage, Eric took the coordinates and recorded them and Charlie and Hazel fixed up the cabin shelter with a hastily cut ridgepole over which a tarp was stretched. Then they gathered some fresh evergreen boughs for a thick, warm, pleasant-smelling carpet. The old rusty stove was still useable and Charlie unearthed the equally rusty stovepipes, which he connected. After cutting a hole in the tarp with his knife, he thrust them through the hole.

"Won't it catch fire?" Jason asked.

"No, it'll just melt around it a bit, then it will be okay," Charlie replied.

Sometime during the last winter, Charlie had travelled here by snowmobile and built a heavy log cache about fifty metres from the cabin, and stored some equipment and a large assortment of food ready for this trip. He had fastened the log cache by nailing long spikes through the logs to ensure that it was secure. He now came to tell us the dismal news that a grizzly bear had torn the logs from the door, logs that were twenty-five centimetres in diameter, and eaten all the food supplies. Then out of pure orneriness, it had chewed the gas cans, spilling out gas and oil, and then crunched up kettles and pans. Nothing edible or usable was left.

Jason was in agony with his ankle and it was quite swollen. Continuing to walk on it for a few kilometres after he had twisted it had exacerbated the injury so he took some painkillers to alleviate his pain. I discussed the injury with him and Eric, and we looked at the alternatives facing us. We could wait where we were for a few days with hardly any food and see if the ankle would heal enough for Jason to walk for another five or six days to Fort Ware. Or Eric could call a helicopter with his satellite phone and fly Jason out that night—that is, if a helicopter could reach us from its base, and get to Fort Ware before dark. Otherwise, they could make arrangements to fly out the next morning.

This is where it was brought home to me again about the hardships that First Nations people had endured. All they could have done in days gone by was to wait until the injured person recovered, or insist that he drag himself along with the rest of the clan, or leave him behind and hope that he would recover and catch up with them later on. Either way, many of them would go hungry for days while they waited, unless there was game in the area.

Eric finally made the decision to contact a helicopter pilot through the BC Forest Service. Using his satellite phone, he made contact and was told that the Forest Service had a fire patrol helicopter with enough fuel and enough daylight flying time for him to take advantage of. After a quick conference, Eric decided to go with Jason, because they were both relying on the vehicle that they had left at Fort Ware to take them south. We decided to send Goldie back home as well, because he had developed a bad chafe on his injured shoulder and had been unable to carry very much in the last few days. I also packed up my old, wet and heavy hiking boots, and scouted around for things to make my pack lighter. I packed the fly off my tent and my rifle, which was beginning to show signs of rust after being wet for so long, day after day.

A big fire was built near to the cabin, to help warm and dry us. Charlie kept finding more big logs that were lying around the cabin site, and throwing them on the fire, which was soon roaring. The rest of us, except poor Jason, who watched us with a pained expression on his face, cut down brush and removed anything that looked as though it could get sucked up by the updraft from the huge rotors of the helicopter.

Flying by helicopter was always exciting, but it was not without its dangers. At one time, I thought I would like to take flying lessons in a fixed-wing aircraft, but I found it virtually impossible to decipher the voice that was coming over the radio even when I was a passenger, and I was very aware that whenever anything went wrong with my car it was always a relief to pull over to the side of the road and call a tow truck. What would I do if there was engine trouble in a plane flying at three thousand feet or more? The helicopter pilot had to have a fine touch where the controls must feel like an extension of himself. I thought that I could probably master that part, but technical instruments were beyond me.

A visiting doctor to Fort Ware travelled with Northern Thunderbird Air when he made his twice-monthly visits, then because of timing problems around his clinic appointments in Prince George he decided to visit Fort Ware and Ingenika using a helicopter. He purchased a really small two-seater helicopter. Stopping to fuel up in Mackenzie and then following Williston Lake and the winding logging roads he would arrive in Fort Ware, set the machine down close to the Health Centre, wrap it up with a light nylon cover to keep any snow or rain off and plug the engine heater in. Then with the assistance of the federal Health Nurse and the Community Health Worker he would hold a very busy clinic. Early the next morning he would uncover the helicopter and after warming the engine he would whisk his way south either to Ingenika or back to Prince George to continue his routine visits to the hospital and his clinical duties in his busy medical practice. This schedule went on very successfully. For a while.

One Friday in January, when the temperature hovered around minus twenty-eight degrees Celsius with a cold north wind blowing, the doctor had taken the cover off his helicopter, packed his few bags inside and shortly afterwards he was flying south. In the village, children made their way to school and the Band office opened up. Barely halfway through the first cup of coffee, the phone call came that stopped everything.

Air-Sea rescue in Victoria in southern British Columbia had picked up an ELT (Emergency Locator Transmission) from a downed helicopter somewhere south of Fort Ware. Although there was no local radio station in Fort Ware, the truckers' road radio soon had nearly all the residents aware of the accident.

Without any real coordinator, people rallied around. One man—Charlie Boya—located a young man who had recently taken a guiding and first aid course and he set off down the Finlay River on his snowmobile to search. Donny Van Somer and several other men started to drive down the Russell logging road at the same time the RCMP were starting to drive north on the Russell from Tseh Keh, eighty kilometres to the south. A small plane that was stationed at Finbow (Buffalo Head logging camp) prepared to take off to begin an aerial search.

Word was received by the RCMP of the probable location of the downed helicopter. It was close to where Donny Van Somer was searching and he was notified on the road radio. He radioed for someone with first aid training to head in his direction in case help was needed. He said later that he was not looking forward to finding the helicopter if it had plunged into the ground.

Everyone waited quietly and patiently. Then Donny's voice came over the radio speakers in every vehicle in the area: "I can see the helicopter now. It's on the road and ... and the doctor is getting out, and walking towards me!"

Everyone sighed with relief and hurried to tell the other people the good news. As one Tseh Keh resident said, "It's good to know that the one doctor who cares for us was maybe down but he's not out!" We heard that the carburetor on the helicopter had iced up and the doctor had been able to land on a side road. When he came down, the force of the landing had activated the ELT.

Later on in the year, the doctor resumed flying into the village with his helicopter, and brought his wife on what was to be his last trip by helicopter. What happened afterwards was related to me by several people.

After the clinic at the Health Centre, the doctor and his wife flew southwest to visit some friends at an isolated lodge. As they approached the lodge, flying over a large lake, the engine stalled and the helicopter plunged into the water. The doctor extricated himself from the rapidly sinking machine and came to the surface but he could not see his wife. Fearing that she was still in the cockpit he dove down towards the helicopter but he could not see her. She had managed to undo her seat belt and get out and she surfaced as her husband was swimming down to rescue her. The people at the lodge soon had them both in a boat and back at the lodge where they were dried off. For future trips to Fort Ware, reason prevailed and after that crash, the doctor's wife refused to let her husband travel in anything other than a plane with Northern Thunderbird Air.

It had always been difficult to find a doctor who was willing to give up a few days from a busy practice to visit Fort Ware. I had asked one Prince George doctor if he was willing to visit and he was quite enthusiastic—at least until he told me that he had discussed it with his wife and she was adamant that he not risk his life flying off into the bush to look after some people who had a rather bad reputation. After drawing a blank in Prince George, I was able to negotiate with a doctor from Fort St. John, many miles to the southeast of Fort Ware, to provide a medical service but after about a year he moved to Vancouver Island and I was left searching again.

At Burn Cabin, the rain finally stopped and the clouds began to roll away as we all waited, lost in our own thoughts. Suddenly we heard the steady throb of the Jet Ranger helicopter churning towards us and soon spotted it flying low over the trees. It circled once while the pilot made sure of his landing place, then he brought it in over the cleared area and set it gently down. The downdraft from the rotors whisked smoke and ashes from the still-blazing fire, and Charlie quickly propped an old piece of plywood in front of the fire to prevent any more embers from blowing into the bush, or worse still, into the cabin.

We said hurried farewells, helped Jason into the helicopter, then loaded his and Eric's packs, Goldie, the rifle, and other odds and ends that we thought we could do without, then hurriedly backed away as the pilot increased the engine's power. We watched as it slowly lifted off and headed south and disappeared over the horizon, then Charlie turned to me and said quietly that we were on our own now, without much grub, no GPS and no satellite phone so he was going down to the river to see if there was anything worth hunting that we could eat. I suspect that he was now glad that everything would depend upon him and he would not be competing with the GPS.

"We'll be okay," he said, as he set off down the trail.

The sky continued to clear, and the rays of the setting sun cast long shadows over the cabin. Silence descended and I felt quite at peace with the world.

Hunger and Thirst

A rifle shot echoed around the camp and Hazel and I waited in anticipation for Charlie to reappear, which he did after about fifteen minutes. He asked me to go with him down to the beaver pond where he had shot a large beaver. I followed him down the trail to where the dead beaver lay on the side of the pond. While Charlie cut a long pole for us to carry the beaver back to camp, I turned the animal over to have a closer look at it.

In trapping terms, this beaver would have been classified as a blanket beaver because it was very big and weighed at least twenty-five kilograms. It had a good coat of fur and when I ran my fingers through the long guard hairs I couldn't help but wonder at the process that had been used years ago to make the top hats that were common amongst the gentry of Europe during the 1800s. These days, it was only the RCMP in the north who wore beaver hats, and the fur used was tanned, leaving the guard hairs visible, not processed like the beaver felt hats of earlier centuries. There has been talk about the RCMP changing to fake fur for their winter hats, which would further decrease the earnings of northern trappers. Turning the beaver over, I ran my fingers over its flat tail, which felt very coarse and scaly. Its feet were webbed and when splayed out they were as big as my outstretched hand. The toes were tipped with long, claw-like nails. As I gazed at the lifeless animal, it suddenly struck me that I was looking at supper.

We tied the beaver's legs fore and aft on the pole and then heaved the pole onto our shoulders. The pole bent in the middle with the weight, and as we walked it bounced up and down, digging the pole into our shoulders. The rough ground made it difficult for us to keep pace with each other and the bounces. At our camp, Charlie soon had the beaver skinned and cut up, and he fed the two dogs a generous portion of meat. This was their first real meal in several days, except for scraps and one or two grouse wings, feathers, and guts, and they now bolted down the meat as though they knew there would not be much chance of getting more in the near future.

Hazel cooked some bannock, which we ate with fried beaver meat. The beaver tail was propped up on a stick in front of the old, rusty woodstove where it slowly roasted and then Charlie and Hazel picked at it with evident enjoyment. I tried a minuscule piece, just to say that I had tried it, but the fatty gristle was not to my liking and I was glad to leave the rest for my hosts. Maybe I just wasn't hungry enough!

I was invited to stay with the Boyas in the tiny cabin instead of setting up my soaking wet tent, and it was a pleasurable change to be able to sit upright and to hang up my wet things inside. I lay on my sleeping bag, which had now dried, smelling the fresh pine scent that the needles under me gave off as they were warmed by the heat from the stove.

Charlie and Hazel seemed more relaxed now that there was only the three of us and I certainly felt comfortable in their company. We lay there in an after-supper lethargy, dozing in the heat, sipping tea periodically, no one having to say anything.

As the evening continued, we talked about our supplies, or the lack of them. Charlie said that a lack of grub was a common thing in Fort Ware in times past. I could remember that Tommy Poole had told me the same thing. Tommy and his wife Eva were Elders in Fort Ware and they had always spent most of their time at their winter cabin up the Finlay River or camping out on their trapline. During one of those winters when the snow had been particularly heavy—"more common in the old days," Tommy had said—he and Eva were a long way from home and had run out of food. Their children were hungry and crying, but all their parents could do was keep everyone moving towards the village. Eva pulled the young children on a small sled and Tommy broke trail in the deep snow with his snowshoes, walking ahead for awhile and then walking back to pack the trail down. All the time, they were hoping that perhaps someone would come by with some food or they might reach a camp, but they

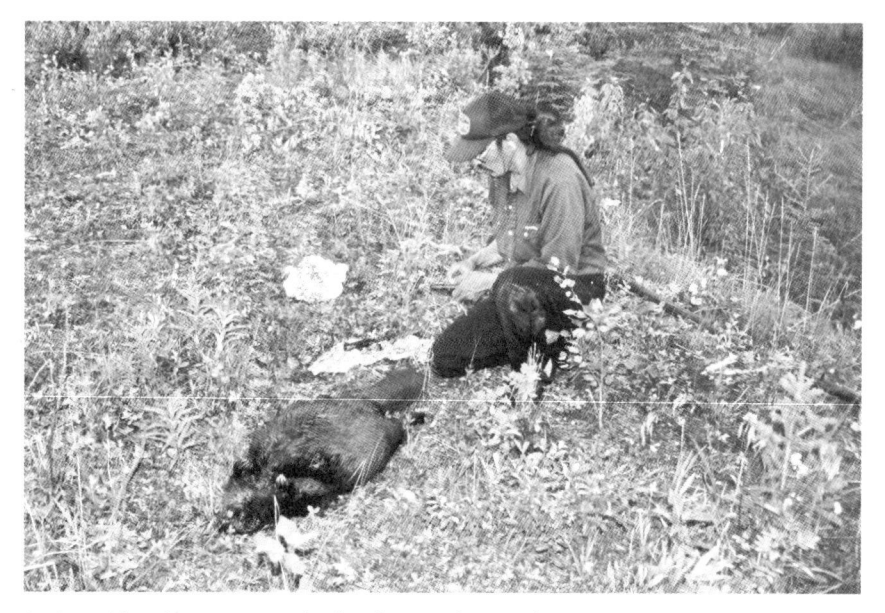

In the midst of lean times, Charlie shoots a beaver for supper. Fresh food at last!

knew it was very doubtful that anyone would be very far from the village because of the bad weather. They stopped and made a big fire and spread some evergreen branches around so that they could stay out of the snow and rest in the warmth of the fire. They did eventually arrive safely in the village, half-starved, but without suffering any ill effects. Eva had said that the worst part of the experience was seeing the children suffer and hearing them cry for some food and being unable to give them anything. This is the sort of background that showed me the stamina and resilience of these mountain people in the face of extreme hardship.

When Williston Lake was first created in the late 1960s, the supply route to Fort Ware was virtually cut off. In the spring flood, when the muddy, log-laden water roared through Deserters Canyon at the mouth of the Finlay River bringing trees and river debris with it, navigation was impossible and planes could not land on floats on the Finlay at Fort Ware for the same reason. (The airstrip was not built until the late 1970s.)

The Finlay River had been the communication link between families who travelled the river to visit one another or to head south in the summertime to work on fire suppression crews or at one of the many sawmills. When river access was cut off, people were unable to visit their relatives south of Fort Ware, and no one could afford to fly out from the village to find work, so people tended to stay in the village, feeling frustrated and powerless to prevent the changes that were happening to their land, their culture and their lives.

When transportation and roads finally improved, local people were not required to haul freight by boat and then man-haul the supplies from the river to the store. Supplies are now shipped in weekly by truck, driven by a non-Native driver, on a four hundred-kilometre gravel logging road from Mackenzie. The supplies are deposited at the door of the large, new, Band-owned store operated by Northern Stores of Winnipeg. Consequently, these arrangements do not give much in the way of employment to Fort Ware residents.

When work did become available, people had to come to terms with the idea of working for five days a week and taking the weekend off to go hunting and fishing. Their lifestyle had been to go hunting and fishing at any time, and then work for a while to earn a few dollars. The irony of this is that they now have to work for wages so that they can take time off to go hunting and fishing which they had the freedom to do at any time previously.

Employers, including the Fort Ware Band, now need workers they can rely on to be on the job all day and to be there at least five days a week. The Band tries to hire as many of its members as it can, and the Band office and the Aatse Davie School are now doing a remarkable job in running their own affairs.

These days the Canadian government provides financial aid to those in need. Therein lies a problem: defining those who are "in need." The Sekani culture has traditionally been one of sharing what you have with those who are without. For example, when a moose was shot, the best pieces of meat would go to the old people, and extended family members would also get a share. Some men are good hunters, and some are content to wait and see what comes their way without hunting.

I approached the Department of Indian Affairs once to ask them to consider the high cost of food in Fort Ware when they allocated funds to the Band for social assistance. I was told that the people in Fort Ware could go and hunt moose to supplement their funds, but when I asked if similar people living on the coast were told to go and catch fish to supplement their income, I could not get an answer. This was when gas prices in Fort Ware were half as much again as gas prices in Prince George, and the welfare payments did not meet the needs of the handicapped or single mothers whose circumstances kept them in the village.

In 2007, Chief Emil McCook retired and Donny Van Somer was elected Chief. This young entrepreneur worked with BC Hydro and Kemess Mines to right some of the problems of the past and the financial compensation received should now help the Band surge ahead. Already the village is showing many improvements.

In a number of books we can read that in the early days of exploration, men from different ethnic backgrounds worked extremely hard and suffered many privations, so that when they came into town where they could relax, they let loose with liquor and then fights often ensued. The ever-present knives and guns—the tools of hunters and trappers—were unfortunately sometimes used to settle arguments.

The Native people must have learned well from those days. After fighting the elements for days and weeks on a trapline or after hunting for food for their families, often nearly starving in the process, they would come to the trader in the village to exchange furs for supplies and goods. Then they would go home and make a batch of homebrew to celebrate and relax with. Some of the people would end up fighting each other when they had drunk too much. Perhaps this form of relaxation was also encouraged by outsiders, who delighted in selling hard liquor at inflated prices. There is no doubt in my mind that liquor affects many First Nations people more severely and much faster than it does non-Aboriginals.

The outlook of people from Fort Ware has not changed very much from the old days except that now, instead of letting off steam after being out on the trail for months, they let off steam because of a feeling of being caged up in the village. There have been some violent confrontations in the village and each time alcohol was the root cause. One young man in his mid-twenties became very jealous of his wife and, after some heated words, he shot and killed her, then he barricaded himself in his house. It took the RCMP several hours to reach Fort Ware. Four of them approached the house to apprehend the perpetrator, but he held them off by threatening to shoot anyone who came close. In a show of bravado, he shouted out that if they shot him, "he would take one or two of them with him." After hours of impasse, he finally came to the door. At least one Mountie had the man in his rifle crosshairs, but as the alcohol wore off, the man finally gave in and was taken into custody without any more bloodshed.

Of course there are family squabbles as there are in any society, but sometimes feelings are exacerbated by inner frustrations and feelings of helplessness. In days gone by, according to Samuel Black, it was acceptable for a woman to wail and scream at her husband and to act in this way when a child died, but the child's father was expected to be unmoved and stalwart. If he had been an Englishman, we would have said that he had to have "a stiff upper lip." Alcohol has broken that cultural more and men now react with tears, anger and bottled-up fury at times.

When the Fort Ware School was administered by the Department of Indian Affairs, it had quite a difficult time recruiting teaching staff, and there was a large turnover of teachers every year. Then, out of the blue, a group of Roman Catholic nuns said that they were willing to provide staff for the school. A group of four teachers, one nun who seemed to act as the cook and cleaner for the group and, surprisingly, a fully trained nurse, arrived in Fort Ware. When the Federal Health Director heard this, I was told to hire her immediately (this occurred when I was working for the Federal Health Department as a nursing supervisor). After this, the Health Centre was renamed the Fort Ware Nursing Station. Sister Anne Laberge was a kindly lady who spent many hours looking after the sick. Even though I told her to try and work within normal working hours, I know that she responded to all calls, serious or not, at any time of the day or night. Sister Anne did not care about the money because she had taken a vow of poverty and her wages went to the church, but she never claimed for any overtime in all the years that she was there.

All went well for several years. Then, after one young man had been drinking heavily, he went to the nuns' residence wielding a large knife, entered the building and threatened the nun who acted as the school principal. She remained calm and was able to talk her way out of the situation, but she was extremely upset by the incident. She clearly felt that the situation arose because the man was angry about something that had happened in school and that the man was very intoxicated. She felt things would calm down afterwards but when the RCMP were informed about it, the perpetrator was removed from the village, charged and placed in custody. Everyone thought that it was all over but when the Bishop heard what had happened he removed the whole group of nuns, including "our" nurse, from the village in spite of their pleading to stay. Fortunately for the village, other staff were recruited for the school and a nurse was hired who came along with her husband who provided moral, if not physical, support for her.

Years later, when I was the Band Manager, I was called one evening by the Community Health Representative to a spousal feud after a couple had aired their grievances about each other while they shared some homebrew. In anger, the man had thrown a heavy cup at his wife with considerable force. Then, seeing that his spouse was bleeding heavily from a head injury, he had taken off in his truck for Tseh Keh, seventy kilometres south. Meanwhile the victim of this onslaught was bleeding profusely from a cut on her forehead and some friends who came by told her to hold a cloth over the wound while they sought medical help. The patient held a towel against her wound but did not apply any pressure and consequently the towel was soon soaked in blood. There wasn't a nurse or doctor in Fort Ware at the time, but there was a doctor in Tseh Keh (Ingenika). When a message was relayed to him by the Heath Representative, he told her that the patient would have to get a ride down to the clinic there. The patient refused to do this, because her spouse was now down there and she was mad at him. Neither pleading, cajoling or threatening did anything to change her mind. I was called to see if I could persuade her to go. I tried, and had the same results as family and friends.

"*You* can do it," she said, pointing at me, "but I'm not going down there!" She thumbed in the general direction of Tseh Keh.

When he heard about this, the doctor said that if that was the case it was okay with him if I sutured the patient. Since the patient was not willing to move, I went to the clinic with the Community Health Representative and gathered the necessary supplies. We went back to the house where the woman was still sitting holding the bloody towel but was now applying pressure as instructed.

When I started to clean the wound, it started bleeding profusely again and I had to get the Health Representative to apply some pressure to it while I prepared the suturing material. The patient didn't even flinch as I injected some local anaesthetic around the wound. I located the bleeder and put a fine catgut suture through it and tied it off, then put half a dozen fine sutures in the laceration to close the wound. When I had cleaned up, she asked for a mirror and looked quite pleased with what I had done. I could just imagine her pointing it out to her spouse and saying: "Just look at what you did to me!"

Again, and as usual, the couple were together again when I saw them next and the visiting nurse had removed the sutures. I wanted to look at the healed physical wound but I thought that it might open up old psychological wounds between the couple, so I never had the opportunity to see the results of my handiwork. When I was asked to do some of these medical procedures, I had to admit that I enjoyed the infrequent forays into what had been common practice in my previous job.

In 1985, an article appeared in the *Vancouver Sun* newspaper entitled "The People of the Mountaintops." In the article, a well-known writer, Terry Glavin, described the northern Sekanis of Kwadacha and Ingenika as:

> the last of B.C.'s hunter-gatherers, who [live] deep in the bush, as isolated as any Indian culture in Canada. Their children learn to hunt and chew snuff at an early age, and schooling is often a trapline tutor on a snowmobile.

> In December that year, a fourteen-year-old boy from Kwadacha (Fort Ware) was with his father at their trapline cabin, fifteen kilometres from the village, when a white gas camp stove that was being repaired late at night, exploded, severely burning the father. The young boy snowshoed back to the village on his own to get help, travelling in the dark, with the temperature hovering around minus thirty degrees. The environment in which the Sekani live has given nearly all of them great stamina and an inherent survival instinct.

The way of life of the Sekani has resulted in some worrisome statistics and the number of people who have been shot or stabbed in Fort Ware is higher per capita than in any other village in British Columbia. Guns and knives are as common in a Fort Ware household as computers are in a southern household, and they seem to be used just as often. They are still the tools of their trade, and young children soon learn to handle these items in their pursuit of meat and furs. As I worked around the village, I soon became accustomed to seeing both young boys and girls skillfully using chainsaws and wielding axes, and outside of the village they could shoot a gun better than many adults from the south.

In all the years that I worked at Fort Ware, I was never threatened and never felt unsafe. The people were generous and friendly, and if an interest was taken in the people or their land, they gladly provided any information that was requested.

Listening to the triumphs and the tragedies of Fort Ware as we lay on the aromatic evergreen branches in our shelter, far away from modern distractions, it was easy to picture what Hazel and Charlie told me. I hoped I would remember all these thoughts and concerns that were expressed to me when I returned to my home in Prince George. Whenever possible, I made notes in my diary, usually by the light of a small headlight that I carried, although when I had been in my tent there was enough light to write by.

The sky was now clear, and the moon, which was just over the first quarter, appeared from behind a high mountain. This was 2,743-metre Mount Cushing in the Thudaka Range to the southwest. After all the activity of the day, and what felt like an intrusion into our little bit of backwoods by the helicopter and all that it represented, the natural peace of the trail now again enveloped us. I slept soundly that night, comfortable in my corner of the cabin—that is, until very early in the morning when I woke up hearing my name called rather insistently.

"Keith!" There it was again, "Keith!" I was instantly awake, thinking we were about to be attacked by a bear, and the thought rushed into my mind that I hadn't got a rifle anymore.

Baby Lakes

Charlie was sitting up on his sleeping bag. When he saw me sit up, he said quietly, "Oh, that's good! I couldn't hear you breathing so I went across to you and watched you really closely for thirty-five minutes (he meant seconds, I'm sure). I couldn't see or hear you breathing, and I was worried!"

Because in Charlie's estimation, I was a relatively old man, he had been worrying about my health and safety all along. He realized that I had been exerting myself much more than I usually did, and he was apparently expecting me to kick the bucket any time. Yet he hadn't suggested that I go with the others in the helicopter—something I would have refused to do anyway.

I looked at my watch and saw that it was five o'clock. I couldn't help smiling to myself after he had explained waking me up, then he said, "It's okay, you can sleep longer now!" I thought that if I had woken up suddenly and saw Charlie's face a few centimetres away, peering intently at me in the half-light, I might have fulfilled his expectations and had a heart attack. It was impossible to go back to sleep with all the adrenaline still coursing through my veins, so I just lay there and dozed on and off for another hour.

Later in the morning, we cleaned up around the cache and Charlie tried to repair the log door, straightening and reusing the large spikes. He put all the cardboard from the ripped boxes, the chewed up food cans and all the other debris that the bear had left, into a big pile and made a bonfire of it. When the fire had burned itself out, we packed up and the three of us left with the two remaining dogs. My pack felt much lighter without the things I had sent back to Fort Ware.

The trail now had a bit of everything for us—downed trees, soft moss up to our knees, swamps to slosh through. Later in the day I could smell horses, which I thought was very unusual out here. Almost immediately we saw a muddy horse trail heading west, off towards our right, and Charlie surmised that a hunting guide had taken a few head of horses from Fort Ware to an outfitters camp at Johiah Lake. The trail was really churned up and we soon had black mud smudged all the way up our pant legs. Charlie said that one year, farther up the Trench, some horses had lived in the wild up by the Frog River, and had even bred there, but the harsh winters and the wolves finally finished them all off. The snow had been so deep that the horses could not scratch for food and they couldn't run or defend themselves either.

The Kechika had now been reduced from a deep powerful river to a fast-running mountain stream as we neared its source at the top of Sifton Pass. The trail came down to the water's edge and we found an old winter cache of Charlie's that another bear had ransacked. Cans, tarps and boxes were scattered through the surrounding bush.

The weather stayed clear, and we marched on, one foot automatically following the other. I knew that if I stopped it would be hard to get going again but at one point I was impelled to stop to watch a big bull moose run through the trees at great speed, his big plate antlers bending saplings in front of him as though they were straws. A wonderful sight, and of course, my camera was deep in my pack.

My camera, still functioning when I really wanted to pull it out of my pack for something memorable, had been thoroughly abused. It had been wet in the rain, bumped into trees, sat upon and scratched. The flash housing wouldn't snap down any more and I had lost the lens cap, so at this point in the trip I had packed it securely away in the middle of my pack. If I had been inclined to try to dig it out, it would have wasted time and I would also have missed seeing the moose careening through the bush. The picture was etched in my mind instead of on film.

After following a line of tall, grey and gravelly hoodoos, where Charlie said you could usually see sheep although there were none that day, we looked back down the Kechika Valley and could see that we had been gradually climbing. In a clearing on the side of the Kechika River, we made camp on a gravel bar just below Sifton Pass. We had come fourteen reasonably comfortable kilometres. The weather had cleared up and we enjoyed the last rays of the sun, which turned the mountaintops a beautiful gold. My tent door faced northwest and framed a magnificent view of the Rockies, with evergreens forming a carpet right up to the steep rocky cliffs. In the foreground, the swirling white water of the Kechika gave the finishing touch to the picture.

We ate fried beaver, fried "chicken" that Charlie had shot with his slingshot, and the remains of the bannock from the night before, which added the finishing touch to our meal. I doctored my heels as usual with the red moss and duct tape, noting that the sores were staying clean and looking like they would soon heal, if I could only give them a good rest. A warm campfire reflected in the restless waters of the Kechika River made for an idyllic setting, and gave us a real "Rocky Mountain High."

It rained during the night, and rain continued sporadically throughout the day, at one time coming down in torrents that looked very much like sleet. Fresh snow outlined the tops of the mountains, and a low-lying fog surrounded the bases, but towards the end of the day both snow and fog melted away and the sun struggled at last to show itself before disappearing behind the mountains again.

We had breakfast consisting of a Bisquick pancake made from a small packet I had found in the bottom of my pack—that, and a cup of black coffee, and we were ready for the trail again. Charlie thought that we should be able to make it to Fox Lake. He was hoping that there would be some supplies at his cabin there, although he was now worried about the behaviour of the bears, which, he said soon learned to associate cabins with easy food. With the last two caches destroyed by bears, he was already anticipating a destroyed and foodless cabin.

By lunchtime we had reached Baby Lakes, where two small lakes were joined at the isthmus by a thick island of willows. I had been here in the wintertime, travelling by snowmobile, when the snow had literally been chest high. I had ridden out into the middle of the lake on my snowmobile and then made the mistake of stopping. The snowmobile wouldn't move ahead, so I jumped off with the idea of pushing it and then jumping on, but when I jumped off I seemed to keep going down and down into the soft powder, and when I finally reached bottom I couldn't reach up to the snowmobile handlebars. I spent half an hour trying to swim ahead in the snow, so that there was some base on which the snowmobile could get a purchase. It finally worked, but as usual I was soaking wet with sweat by then, even though it was twenty degrees below zero.

I had thought that the lakes were named because of their small size, but now I learned that the northernmost Baby Lake was a traditional camping spot and we found a clearing in the trees overlooking the east side of the lake. Apparently, at a winter camp many years ago, a family had been camped here in bitterly cold weather and their baby had died. The parents couldn't do anything with the little body and were too far from any village, so they did what the Carrier people did. They wrapped up their infant and placed it on a platform in the trees to keep animals from disturbing it. No one seems to know any other details, but as I listened to the story I couldn't help but cast my eyes around the trees that surrounded us. Of course, after this length of time, there wasn't anything left. New trees would have grown up to replace the dead ones. Still, it was impossible not to look around at the trees and though I couldn't see anything, my imagination filled out the picture quite adequately.

I had been in this area a few years ago with Craig McCook and Charlie Boya when they were hunting moose in the wintertime. The lakes had really good moose feed in the willows and red osier dogwoods that surrounded the lakes and the numerous moose tracks we saw verified that it was a popular place. Craig suddenly stopped his snowmobile and pointed ahead. Two moose were grazing, but even as we stopped they caught our scent and ran up and over a small hill. Craig quickly donned his snowshoes and grabbed his rifle and headed off around the side of the hill. Charlie and I waited by our machines, not wanting to be mistaken for a moose. About fifteen minutes later, we heard two shots and before the echo had died away another shot rang out. Craig reappeared, calmly smoking a cigarette. He told us he had shot the two moose, who had crossed the hill and must have thought they were safe. A real bushwhacking event!

We drove our snowmobiles over to where the two moose were lying about twenty metres apart. Craig and Charlie immediately started to butcher them. Apart from the smell and the blood and guts, it was a pleasure to watch these two men at work. The hide was carefully cut off and laid in the snow with the hair side down, then both animals were deboned and the meat placed on the hide. The ribs were placed on top of the pile of meat and the hide was wrapped around it all. Using his sharp sheath knife, Craig made holes around the perimeter of the hide, through which he wove a piece of yellow nylon rope. The rope was pulled tight so that the whole

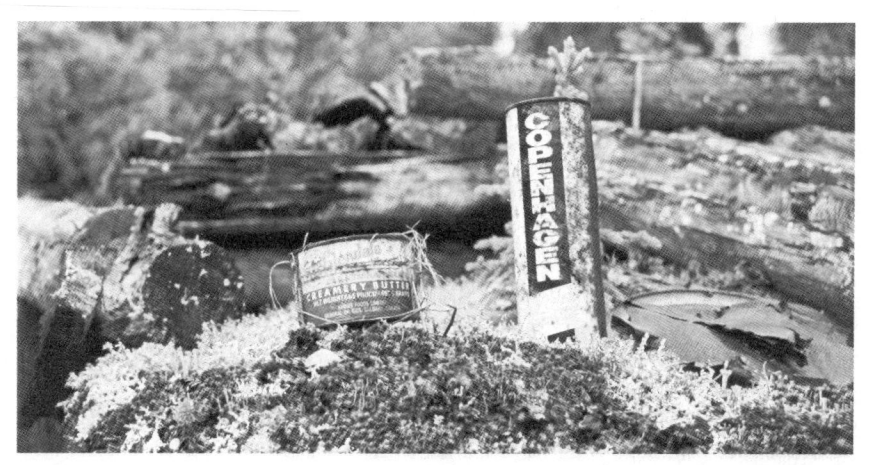

Some artifacts from the 1960s found in the cabin, including a Copenhagen tobacco tin.

package was brought together like a huge purse string. This is how the old-timers transported meat to their camps before there were any toboggans. The hide soon froze and with the hair lying the right way, a heavy load could be transported quite easily over the snow.

We were going to haul the meat back to Fort Ware behind a snowmobile. Because Craig had a powerful short-track machine that caused the track to dig itself into the deep snow when he tried to pull the "moose sled," it was decided that I would have the honour of pulling the load behind my long-track Tundra. When everything was ready, the two men gathered up all the bones, the offal and other bits and pieces and put them in the well of a spruce tree (a hole around large trees where the snow has either melted or been sheltered by overhanging branches). Once this was done, snow was kicked over it all and Craig said something about not wanting bad weather. I was reminded of my experience with the two young men from Fort Ware when we were on the logging road with the moose I had killed with my sheath knife. I assumed that this was another example of the same cultural belief.

I towed that package of moose meat all the way to Fort Ware without it breaking open or coming undone. The only near mishap occurred when I was crossing a narrow creek and my snowmobile broke through the ice just as I reached the far bank. Between us, we were able to haul the machine out of the water followed by the moose sled and then I was able to continue on my way.

After we left Baby Lakes, we travelled down the Davie Trail for a few hours. We stopped on the south side of Sifton Pass in a grassy clearing where

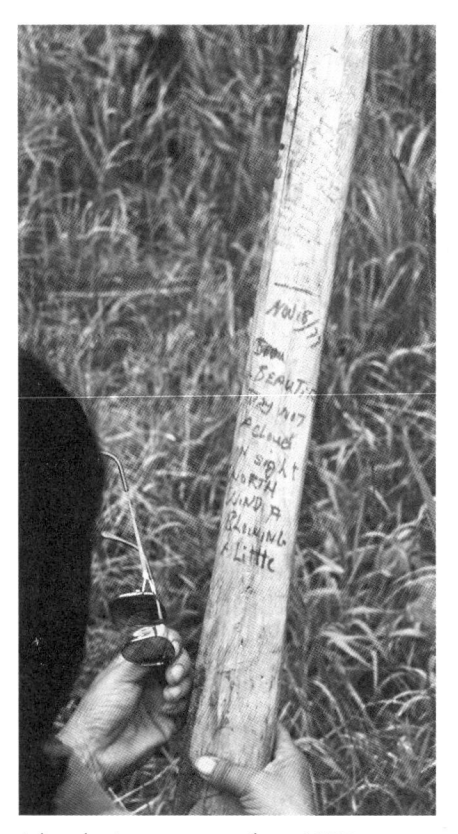

A handwritten message from 1977 on a marten stretcher board.

there was an old cabin that had belonged to old John McCook, Hazel's father. Hazel herself had spent a portion of her teenage years at this cabin and the location held something special for her.

According to a handwritten notice inside the door, the small cabin had been built in October 1958. It had been built of unpeeled logs that had now almost been peeled by the elements and insects, and the old logs were almost black. The roof was made of ingenious alternating scoop logs, where the logs had a "V" cut out of the whole length, then they were placed on the roof with another series of scoop logs inverted on top of them with the "V" facing downwards so that the rain would drain off the cabin roof. Moss was beginning to take over the roof and as often happened to these old cabins, a small spruce tree had taken root on top, finding some nourishment in the roof.

The small loft was full of sand and gravel, the only fireproof material around. Besides being available in the vicinity of the cabin, it was free and served as insulation in the wintertime when the sand and gravel would retain the heat generated from the stove during the day and would be released during the night when the fire in the stove had gone out.

A narrow doorway with the homemade door still attached led into the single room. Two sapling bedframes were still standing, one on either side of the cabin underneath two sixty-centimetre square windows. The beds had a thick layer of dried grass on them that had once served as mattresses. The remains of a table was nailed to the back wall and a rusted-out metal stove stood in a corner with some collapsed lengths of stovepipe around it. There was the unmistakable smell of pack rats, the new residents. Scouting around, Charlie found an old tin that had held ten packages of Copenhagen tobacco. Its advertising was still legible: "Best Chew Made." This tobacco remains a Fort Ware necessity even today. Another vestige of the past that turned up was an old tin of Glendale Creamery Butter, made in Calgary.

Charlie and Craig, his brother-in-law, had last been at this cabin in 1978, when they had been trapping. A message written on an old marten stretcher board was dated November 18, 1977, and said: "Beautiful day, not a cloud in sight. North wind blowing a little."

The cabin was located in a beautiful peaceful setting, surrounded by old conifers with a backdrop of majestic mountains. I wondered aloud how long it would remain that way. Apparently an exploration company had been in the area north of the pass and had found a rare mineral called mannardite. If this mineral is mined, the peace at Sifton Pass could soon be shattered—but not if Chief Donny Van Somer of Fort Ware has his way. Donny's position was that no mining should take place on Band land without the Band's permission and involvement. The Band is reluctant to see the land opened up with roads and mining traffic—which have usually had a negative impact on Indian villages.

After a rest at the cabin, we set off again, walking now through tall pine and spruce timber, where the ground was covered with blueberry bushes. The purple fruit looked very inviting. At the risk of getting left behind, Hazel and I stopped periodically to gather a handful or so, which we ate as we walked quickly to catch up to Charlie. He was soon out of sight, though, in a hurry to reach his cabin at Fox Lake.

The trail was easy to see and in good condition and the closer we got to Fox Lake, the more frequent were the tree blazes. A welcome sight was the rippling water of Fox Lake showing brightly through the trees. The Fox River ("Noohsehe Ts'eli" literally means "Fox River") runs out of the south end of the lake. According to one authority on BC place names, the Fox River was named for William Fox, the manager of the Hudson's Bay store at Fort Grahame at the end of the nineteenth century. Whether the First Nations people adapted that name to their own language or whether it was a coincidence is not now known. Fox Lake was where Charlie Boya had built a cabin as his second home, close to John and Minnie McCook's old cabin. Now, as Hazel and I approached the cabin, we let ourselves think and talk about food supplies again.

Fox Lake

We followed a dry, high trail along the east shore of the lake and then climbed the hill to the cabin, which was located on a small bay at the southeast end of the lake. It had been built on a hillside, snuggled into a natural hollow where there was a good view of Fox Mountain to the southwest, and almost the whole length of the lake could be seen. The cabin was built of unpeeled logs with a sod roof. Grass could be seen growing in tufts on top of the building. The windows had been covered with boards for protection from the bears that usually prowled around in the summertime but we could see that the boards had already been removed by Charlie and were lying around on the ground.

Charlie was muttering about "those damned bears." Clearly a bear had also ransacked this cabin, getting in through the small unprotected window beside the door on the porch. Seemingly becoming disoriented inside the cabin, it had thrashed around, throwing furniture and cupboards hither and yon. It had found a cache of food in the cabin that had been stored in 45-gallon steel barrels, and it had devoured or spoiled nearly everything. Fortunately, Hazel had secreted a small amount of bannock flour for such emergencies that the bear hadn't found. Later she and Charlie went up the hillside and picked huckleberries to add to an oven bannock she was planning to make.

Fox Lake 227

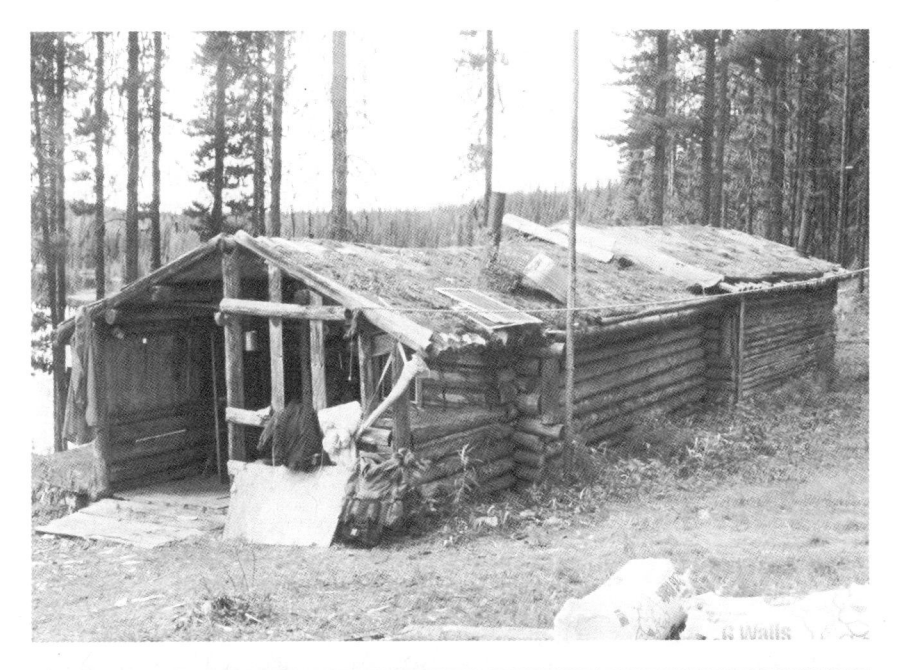

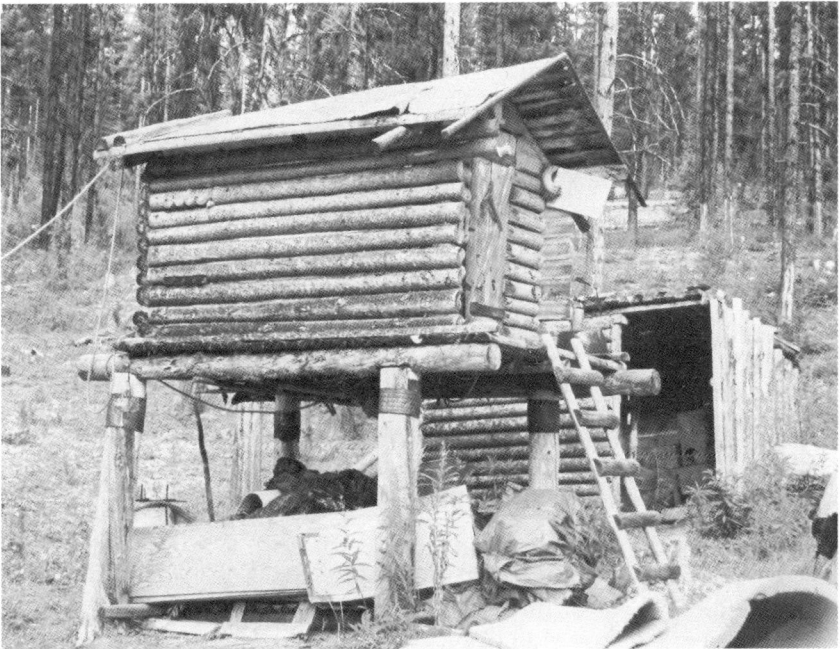

The Fox Lake cabin (top) and the Fox Lake cache (below) had both been ransacked by bears before the hikers arrived.

Charlie and Hazel started to clean up the cabin. When I started to help, Charlie suggested I look after my feet instead. He brought a tub of very warm water over to me, where I was sitting on a soft roll of plastic wrapped insulation. He poured some salt into the water and told me to soak my feet. I was surprised that the bear had not found the salt. I sat with my feet in the tub and felt that this was the pampering of a kind that I could get used to really easily! With another fifteen kilometres behind us, my feet were glad of the special care.

While Charlie and Hazel were away picking berries, I walked over to the cabin, and ducking my head, I entered the small doorway. Over the years the cabin had settled, not having been built on any foundation, and as the foundation logs softened, so the cabin sank, and the doorway was now only about 1.5 metres high. The cabin looked exactly like a trapper's cabin should, with low log beams and some fur stretcher boards jammed into several corners. A rusting but useable tin woodstove sat in one corner by the door. Behind it was a stack of split pine firewood, and on the stove sat a large fire-blackened cooking pot filled with water. A handmade table stood against the side wall, covered with a sheet of linoleum. The seating was made of rounds of logs with small pieces of carpet tacked to the top of them.

One of the fascinating things about this cabin was the writing on the walls, left by unknown authors. This was not the crude writing you see in some urban graffiti, but the sort that can pique your interest and draw you to add your own name to the growing list of backcountry adventurers who have visited the cabin. In this regard, the cabin at Fox Lake was not unique. Cabins all over the north have their walls plastered with messages that record comings and goings. Certainly this would not be tolerated in most urban homes, but wilderness cabin walls serve as ongoing message boards, giving times and dates of arrival and departure that are the equivalent of any public transportation schedule.

These messages are written with felt pens, pencils, and pieces of charcoal from the woodstove. In one old cabin on a northern riverbank, someone painstakingly cut out letters from a box of Aunt Jemima Pancake Mix and glued them (one would assume with the pancake mix) to the log wall—to let others know that they had stayed at the cabin during a storm, and had a lot of time on their hands. Old calendars, pages torn out of notebooks, pieces of cardboard boxes, and the logs themselves, all provide surfaces on which to leave a message. One shelter I stayed in was festooned with miniature carved canoes and paddles on which the names of modern-day voyageurs had been written. Unique models of mosquitoes, all with names and addresses and even telephone numbers on them, were hung at another place by hard-bitten (pun intended!) summer visitors who were proud to have survived the hordes of mosquitoes in the area. In Charlie's cabin, a homemade mosquito danced above the heat of the stove, its egg carton body and purple feathered wings reminding us of the reality of summer bush living.

As I looked around, I saw the name Colin, the Fort Ware store manager. Periodically he would take a few days off and go visit one of the camps, and I made a trip to Fox Lake with him once in the wintertime. One spring, he and I planned to visit Charlie Boya's camp at Fox Lake. Colin could not leave until after the store closed and it was dark, but the snowmobiles had lights, so we decided to leave as soon as we had eaten. We packed extra gas on the machines and a few clothes and some food and set off through the village. Colin dropped his glove and circled around to get it, scooping it off the snow as he zoomed by. Somehow his thumb was caught under the track and it was twisted severely as he tried to yank his hand away. We stopped and I looked at his hand in the light from the still-running snowmobile. The joint of his thumb was swollen and painful but he could move it without any trouble and he said he still wanted to go on, so off we went into the darkness. Every time we stopped, he massaged his thumb and said that holding the snowmobile throttle was the hardest part.

We arrived at the Fox Lake cabin late at night and were welcomed by Charlie and Hazel. The small cabin was almost covered with snow that blew up to the cabin site from the lake below and deposited itself in the lee of the cabin until eventually the whole hillside was a sheet of hard-packed snow. The advantage of this was that the cabin was virtually draft free; the disadvantage was that when Charlie reached the cabin for the first time after freeze-up, he had to dig away the huge snowdrift from the cabin so that he could find the door and then shovel snow from around the chimney before he could light a fire in the cookstove.

Colin and I unrolled our sleeping bags and eyed the one spare single bed. "Toss you for it," Colin said.

"Okay." I replied, not relishing the thought of sleeping on the wood floor—but if I had to, so be it. "Tails!" I called out, as the coin flipped into the air. We both glanced at the coin on the back of Colin's hand. As I laid my sleeping bag out on the bed, I said, "I guess today is not your lucky day. I hope your thumb will be comfortable resting on the wooden floor!"

The next morning was a brilliant day with the sun shining in a cloudless sky. I was looking forward to the journey back. Colin decided to stay another day at the cabin so I loaded up. Only then did I realize that with leaving after dark the previous night, I had neglected to bring my sunglasses. Usually Hazel had a spare pair in the cabin, but she searched all over without finding any.

I set off. Fortunately much of the trail was in the trees, but on the lakes and creeks I had to pucker up my eyes like a couple of old prunes. I did not get snowblinded, but when I opened the door of the house I was staying in at Fort Ware it seemed oppressively dark until my eyes adjusted some time later.

Travelling north of Fort Ware was always exciting because there were no roads, no logging and no people. The country was unspoiled and in the wintertime there was a palpable silence. When travelling on foot or by snowmobile, there was an element of danger and you had to rely on yourself for survival. I shuddered at the idea of a road or railway corridor through the Trench or worse still the flooding of this valley for hydroelectric power generation. The logging road to Fort Ware in the 1990s was progress enough.

It was now hard to picture the exterior of the cabin since it had been covered in snow in the wintertime, but the interior was virtually the same. In many well-used cabins throughout Canada's northland, the owners leave grocery lists pinned to the wall or they leave lists of supplies that have been taken to other cabins or that are needed later. Descriptions of what the weather has been like, and the highs and lows of different trips are all there to read.

On a winter skiing trip to a BC provincial park, my wife and I came to a wardens' cabin where an official notice warned people to "KEEP OUT!" It was affixed next to the door, which we found to be loosely fastened with a smashed padlock. Since the cabin had already been entered, we looked inside, where everything was still neat and tidy. In the visitor's book on the table, we saw that the warden had written: "Now that you are in the cabin, please make sure that you shut the door behind you when you leave." Since the isolated cabin had obviously been broken into before, why had they bothered to padlock the door again, which would now have to be repaired? And why leave a visitor's book inside?

Visitors to these remote cabins have traditionally left them in the same condition that they found them—sometimes even better, refilling wood boxes with split wood and kindling, ready for the next needy person.

Even in these days of snowmobiles and four-wheel bikes, very few wilderness cabins are locked up, but those that are have messages written on the outside walls or the cabin door. It seems that trappers, hikers, skiers or pilots all feel that they must leave some communication for others that may pass by that way.

A cabin on an island on one of the Nation Lakes in central British Columbia has served as a shelter for many people who left written glimpses of their visit. One example reads: "May 6. Wind and rain. Left cabin swept, with a supply of wood, with our many thanks. Shored front wall—top half—logs loose. John and Shirley, Vancouver." This cabin was the scene of a tragedy that occurred when other visitors were there from North Vancouver and their story unfolds in daily notes stuck to the cabin wall.

"Aug 2. Wet, cold, welcome cabin, dry, warm. Many thanks, Andy and Robbie."

"Aug 3. Aircraft crashed 2 miles from cabin. 5 pm. Saved pilot—but could not save 2 passengers."

"Aug 4. Rescue aircraft picked up injured pilot, departed early 4 Aug."

"Aug 4, 5, 6. Rescue party for plane. Cabin was great, and clean, few supplies left for next. Grant, Roger, Adair."

"Aug 13. Search party stayed in cabin—left wood & some groceries. Nice spot. Enjoyed by Grant, Jerry, Jack."

Other messages were left by upbeat hunters who just had to tell someone about their prowess, even though weeks might pass before the note would be read by anyone:

"Oct 16. Dick, Don, Ron, Bob. 3 moose + 1 going down to camper."

A message in another lonely cabin was simple and to the point:

"Rudy O'Quinn, Cape Breton. Thank you for the use of cabin."

In Charlie's cabin at Fox Lake I counted over two hundred messages left by visitors who had passed through, and Charlie himself had virtually left a journal of his comings and goings ever since he had built an addition to the cabin in 1972.

Some of the messages in the cabin were more personal but humorous:

"Dionne went to sleep in her soup."

"Fox Lake Hilton. Reasonable rates. Lots of parking." (The nearest road is over one hundred and seventy kilometres away.)

Sometimes you would need to know the cabin owner or his friends if you wanted to decipher who had been at the cabin, since some messages were quite detailed—except for the names of the visitors:

"April 2. 4:05 pm. Windy today. Kinda cold. Hope it turns a little warm. CB, HB, CB, IJB."

Because of storms, or just to rest up, I have spent many hours and days in isolated cabins, without any radio or television, no daily newspaper, and quite often, no one to talk to. When firewood has been cut and split to replace what has been used, and old, usually *very* old, magazines have been read, I never get to the stage where I am climbing the walls—I just go ahead and read them.

Shortly after returning with a big canister of luscious-looking huckleberries and while Hazel busied herself cooking the berries, Charlie went down to the lake to go fishing. Luckily the bear had not broken his fishing pole and the box of lures was still intact. There was an old aluminum canoe down by the shore, and Charlie intended to paddle it out to a favourite spot on the lake that usually provided some good fish. Josh Boya, Charlie's son, had caught a seven-kilogram lake char on this lake, one of many large fish that the lake produced.

The canoe had a large gash in its side, but not wanting to be thwarted, Charlie searched through his ruined cache. He found a can with a small amount of roofing tar in it, then he found an old gnarled pine tree, collected some lumps of hard sap, and boiled it down, adding it to the tar. When it had cooled, he smeared the mixture over the gash and then launched the canoe, sitting well back so that the damaged side was out of the water for most of the time. In spite of his industry, the fish did not cooperate and, after several hours, Charlie gave up without having had even a bite.

In the evening we sat in the cabin on rounds of logs. Charlie relit the woodstove and then surprised me by going out to his small shack behind the cabin and starting up a small generator he had stored away in a tall cache that bears could not reach. As it got progressively darker, he even turned on a few lights. Ah, luxury indeed! "Next time I'll put some grub for us up in the cache too," he exclaimed sadly. As we sat and talked, Hazel suggested that we stay at the Fox Lake cabin for another day to rest our weary bones. I did not need convincing and took two Tylenol to help rest them.

Without me prompting them, Charlie and Hazel started to speak again about the changes that were taking place in Fort Ware. They talked about the houses, and what they used to be like compared to those being built now. Charlie started by saying that the scattering of log cabins that once lined the Finlay River have now evolved into regular three- and four-bedroom houses with R20 insulation and white vinyl siding, and the subdivision has expanded across the peninsula that is formed where the Kwadacha, Fox and Finlay rivers meet. The changes were probably good but the village is just not the same, even though a few old log cabins still occupy the riverbank and give some indication of what the village looked like forty years ago. I interpreted this comment to mean that the village had lost its old character and the new houses did not fit into the environment in the same way. I reminded Charlie that in recent years a few log buildings had been built as a training session, a project that appealed to both the men and women who took the course, as it did to other villagers.

We talked about travel and how float or ski-equipped planes no longer have to rely on the vagaries of the river for landing. Wheeled aircraft can now land on a gravel airstrip; even planes as large as a DC3 have landed. A regular daily scheduled aircraft from Prince George brings mail and passengers, most planes piloted by men and women from Northern Thunderbird Air. Many pilots, like the late Ernie Harrison and Lester Bower, flew bush planes into the area in the "fly by the seat of your pants" era. Lester said he had flown the route so many times at low altitudes that he knew the name of every tree between Fort Ware and Prince George. These pilots hauled dogs, camping and trapping gear, canoes strapped to the planes' pontoons and supplies for every conceivable project. The large office and community hall was built of treated lumber from the south, all of it flown in on a Caribou aircraft chartered out of Inuvik.

Charlie had chartered the old Beechcraft plane himself to take Jonathan, his quadriplegic son, and the rest of his family up to his cabin at Terminus Mountain. He had used the same plane to take building supplies, a wheelchair and a quad bike, cramming them all into the plane. Years ago that wouldn't have been possible, and Jonathan certainly couldn't have travelled to Terminus Mountain.

It was now quite dark in the makeshift cabin and the glow from the stove cast a comforting glow on the faces of Charlie and Hazel. During pauses in the conversation, Charlie stirred the embers with a stick and put another piece of wood in the stove. He would then sit back and start reminiscing again.

It was not only First Nations men and women who still had a difficult life, especially when dealing with the bureaucracy. There were also a few "non-status Indians" living in Fort Ware who were treated like outcasts by the government. One extended family lived in a couple of cabins on the west side of the Finlay River. They were thirty metres from the main village but not officially on the Kwadacha Reserve. It was strange that here in the wilderness there could be a group of cabins surrounded by thousands of hectares of trees but to the government there was a barrier as large as the Berlin Wall not only to keep non-Indians off the land but to try to keep the status Indians on the reserve.

These people who lived off-reserve were not "registered status Indians." This meant that they did not have all the benefits of the reserve residents. They lived exactly as their neighbours did, had lived there all of their lives, had trapped and travelled the same trails and had climbed the same mountains, but somewhere along the line a mother or grandmother had married a non-Native. They lost their status and became "outcasts"—another case of people living on "the other side of the tracks." The Kwadacha Band distributed welfare cheques to local status and non-status Natives alike, with the knowledge and approval of Indian Affairs.

Most of the time life continued day after day. One old man named Frank, who lived off-reserve on the west side of the Finlay River, received his Old Age Pension from the federal government. The high cost of food and fuel ate up all of his monthly cheque, but he could get by with wild meat that was brought to him and his wife by the young members of the family and firewood was close at hand.

Then this seventy-three-year-old man began losing weight and, on some mornings, he couldn't get out of bed. The visiting nurse said that he should go to Prince George for a thorough medical check-up because his symptoms were serious. The cost of a flight to Prince George was three hundred dollars each way, plus there would be food and accommodation requirements for several days and local cab fare from the motel to the hospital. Frank hadn't enough money. The Department of Indian Affairs was approached for assistance but the request was turned down because Frank was not a "status Indian." Frank's wife approached me to tell me that she was worried about her husband's deteriorating condition. I thought the situation very unjust, and after speaking with an official at Indian Affairs and getting nowhere, I spoke to the CBC radio people and the issue was broadcast all over British Columbia. After the story aired, the phone started to ring as offers came in from generous British Columbians pledging to pay for Frank's travel expenses.

Arrangements were made and Frank arrived in Prince George and was helped to a taxi to take him to the hospital where he soon received the necessary care. Unfortunately, in spite of the generosity of people, Frank's medical problem remained but the Department of Indian Affairs was adamant that Frank would have to pay for his own transportation unless he applied to become a status Indian. Official records and certificates were not easily available and neither Frank nor his relatives could understand the need for all the bureaucratic procedures. It was a process I knew could take years because records had to be researched and affidavits sworn through lawyers—by a seventy-three-year-old sick man living in a small log cabin on the wrong side of the river. To illustrate this poor man's reaction to the civilized world after having lived nearly all of his life out in the bush, when I was driving him from the airport to the hospital along a busy road, I noticed he kept on jerking his body over to one side when he saw an oncoming car. I soon realized that he thought we were going to have a head-on crash because the vehicles seemed so close when they passed us travelling at quite some speed. At first I wanted to laugh, then I tried to put myself in his shoes—or I should say moccasins. I could appreciate that after seeing only a few snowmobiles on bush trails, Frank was astounded at the speed and close proximity of cars and trucks on Prince George roads.

In the small cabin at Fox Lake, Charlie, Hazel and I talked about other problems, the courts, the victims and the perpetrators but we didn't come up with any definitive solutions. The cabin became quiet. I don't know what Charlie and Hazel were thinking, but my mind was whirling. I had spent most of the trip imagining what it was like here in the old, old days. Suddenly I was confronted with the more recent hardships faced by these people. Even though I felt powerless, as the representative white man, I somehow also felt guilty for all of the injustices created by those who thought things would be so much better for these poor people if only they were more like us. My mind kept repeating "What if—?" or "If only—."

The next morning, Charlie took the canoe back onto the lake but after an hour he came back up to the cabin empty-handed. I was surprised that he had the patience to fish for as long as he had without catching anything. He was usually so active I couldn't imagine him sitting still watching a line, even for five minutes. After he had given up hope of catching anything, he and Hazel decided to walk back along the trail to the carpet of huckleberries we had seen the day before. Hazel and I had stopped there for about fifteen minutes on the way in and had eaten as many as we could pick. Charlie and Hazel had also picked a pail full of berries there the day before. While they were gone, I went down to the canoe and tried my hand at catching some urgently needed food. I didn't get a bite but my feet had the benefit of fresh air, as I kept both feet up in the canoe and let them sit in the sun.

After the morning's activities, we ended up with a big pail of huckleberries, but no fish. Charlie collected all the debris scattered around the cabin by the bear and built a bonfire. He was ready to declare war on bears. He hammered nails through the window coverings so that bears would be discouraged from clawing at the windows, then he put boards on the ground, under the windows, and the boards had nails through them to keep the bears from standing up by the windows. (Charlie called them "welcome mats"). He said that they might make the bears angry, but they might also keep away from the cabin in the future.

Beaver Pass and the Bedaux Sub-Arctic Expedition

It rained again that night. A steady drizzle was still coming down in the morning so by the time we were ready to leave and Charlie had nailed the windows shut and placed the welcome mats to defend the cabin from any unsuspecting bears, we were already soaking wet. We followed a high ridge for about two hours through park-like countryside with very little bush between the seven-metre trees. There were now two trails that led south. The "top trail" was more direct but would lead us through swamps. The hilly "bottom trail" was drier, but would be more tiring. We took the shorter, wetter trail, since we were already wet through. Fortunately, we found the swamps much drier than Charlie had expected, although we still managed to soak our feet in them and most of our clothes were already wet from the underbrush.

By lunchtime, the rain had eased a bit. As we reached Beaver Pass, we found a small, new-looking cabin standing nestled in the pine trees. It was built of peeled logs that still retained their golden colour. The cabin had been

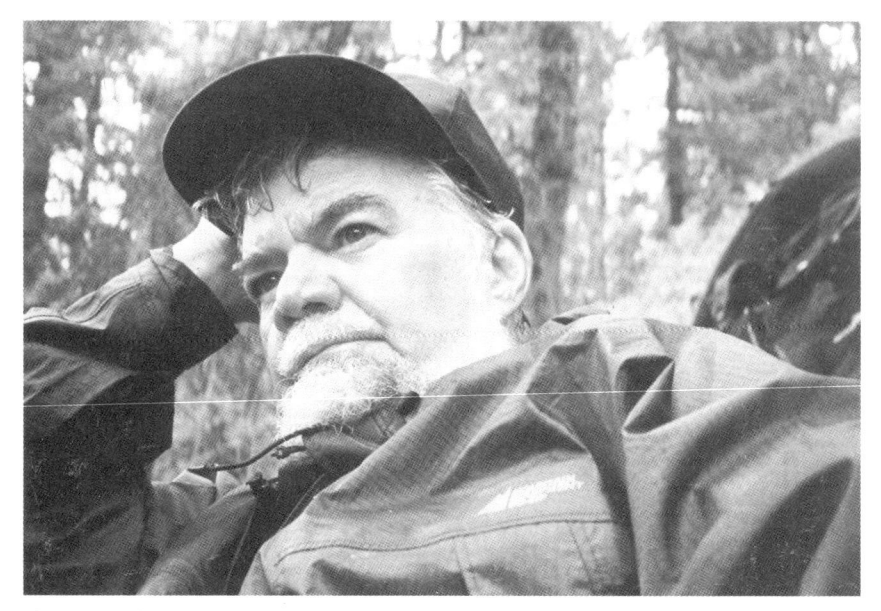

The author feeling exhausted towards the end of the journey.

built on what looked like an esker, a sharp ridge of gravelly soil, with a small lake just below the cabin on one side and the McCook River to the northeast. Very little underbrush grew on this ridge, which was very sandy. I was reminded of a national park with its good trails and minimal underbrush.

Beaver Pass Cabin had been built as a community trails project by young people from Fort Ware in the late 1990s. It was furnished with a small tin woodstove, a table and some rounds of logs for sitting on. Instead of sitting in the shady interior of the cabin, however, we took advantage of the sunshine and tried to dry our clothes and shoes around a small campfire outside.

We found a message on the table in the cabin, written on a scrap of paper by our old friend Annie Charlie from Fort Ware. It said that she and Antoine had been hunting sheep up Burn Mountain with some of their family and that they had left here to head south that morning. After checking the remains of the fire in the stove, Charlie said it looked as though they had been gone longer than a day.

In preparation for crossing more wet sections of trail, a variation of the Fort Ware hip waders came into being when Charlie wrapped his feet, over his socks, in garbage bags, covered everything with duct tape, then slipped his feet once again into his remarkable shoes. Hazel had her own variation: when she changed her socks at lunchtime, she put a large Ziploc bag over each foot!

I saw that my feet and hands were beginning to show signs of swelling. I could pick up the skin on the back of my hand and it would stay puckered up, a sure sign of dehydration. My problem was the scarcity of drinking water. Sometimes it had been pouring all over me as rain, yet I was unable to find anything potable to drink. At times, there wasn't any water to be had anywhere.

A kilometre to the east of Beaver Pass cabin, on an esker overlooking the McCook River, there were three graves. They were now hard to find, having been grown over with ground birch and small aspen trees. Francis Charlie's wife had been buried here—Francis was an Elder of Fort Ware. His wife had died in their cabin in the valley below, perhaps of pneumonia, and long before there were any health services for people who lived in remote areas. In those circumstances, people were buried wherever it was possible. Francis himself had asked to be buried by his wife at this site when he died, but he passed away in springtime just before breakup so it was impossible to accede to his wishes. We considered taking the casket to this site by helicopter or snowmobile, but other family members would not have been able to go. Besides, the cost of a helicopter was prohibitive, the creeks were beginning to break up, and the alternative to the helicopter was to haul the coffin by snowmobile along wet bumpy trails, which would have been very undignified. Old Francis was eventually buried in the cemetery in Fort Ware.

Far below the hill where the graves were, in a clearing by the side of the river, we could see the remains of Francis Charlie's old cabin. The roof had caved in and no one had lived in it for over thirty years. The cabin now belongs to the Charlie family from Fort Ware, but whenever any of the young people visit, they stay at the new cabin at Beaver Pass.

There is a winter trail that leads from the old cabin across the river heading southeast to Weisener Lake, a beautiful long lake nestled right in the Rocky Mountains. Like many of the old trails in the Trench, the Weisener trail is rarely used now.

After a good rest, we continued south down the Davie Trail. From Beaver Pass Cabin, the trail was very unusual. It continued to follow the high ground, as do most trails, but this stretch was almost six metres wide and cut as straight as a die for several kilometres. We were pretty sure that this section of trail had been cut by the Bedaux Sub-Arctic Expedition of 1934, which had gone as far as Sifton Pass before giving up in September of that year.

Charles Eugene Bedaux was born in Paris, France, on October 26, 1887, and went to the United States sometime around 1906. He was evidently a brilliant man, an efficiency engineer who was a leader in the field of scientific management. He became a millionaire, owning several large companies. He was well-known internationally, and hosted the wedding of the Duke of Windsor and Wallis Warfield Simpson at his French Chateau de Candé in 1937.

Bedaux was also a good friend of André Citroen, who was developing tracked vehicles for use in the desert and rough country, and who apparently wanted them field-tested. Depending on which account you read, Bedaux dreamed up a great publicity stunt for the Citroens and thus the "Bedaux Sub-Arctic Expedition" was born. The plan was to find an overland route through uncharted country from Edmonton, Alberta, to Telegraph Creek on the Stikine River in western British Columbia. This was a distance of 2,400 kilometres and resembled the route the Royal Northwest Mounted Police had taken in the eighteenth century.

Bedaux started from Edmonton on July 6, 1934. The real wilderness portion of the trip began at Fort St. John, and it was here that he hired a large number of cowboys and trail-cutters to accompany him. He had an unparalleled entourage with him—reportedly dozens of cowboys and pack horses, and five half-track Citroens. He also took with him two well-known surveyors, Ernest Lamarque and Frank Swannell, who were sent along by the Canadian government. Their job was to map the route the expedition followed.

The trail-cutters' advance party, led by Ernest Lamarque, blazed a trail to the original destination, Telegraph Creek, but the actual trail-cutting finished at Sifton Pass. Lamarque was more of an artist-surveyor than the more mathematical Swannell. He had gone on ahead of Bedaux, travelling with a Kaska man, Jack Stone, drawing scenes with pen and ink. A mountain pass is named after Lamarque and the creek flowing down from the Sifton Pass was named Jackstone Creek. Although I think that the Kaska or Sekani already had names for these creeks, it seems fitting that the creek bore the name of a Kaska man.

After the incomplete expedition ended, some authorities suspected that Bedaux had wanted to map the interior of the province for the Nazis but nothing could be proved. It was peculiar that Swannell's surveying equipment was thrown out by Bedaux because it was too bulky, yet he retained luxury items that could easily have graced a royal banquet. The true intent of the expedition was thus left open to question. Swannell was left with very little in the way of resources to chart the expedition's progress through what was mostly uncharted territory, but he still dutifully recorded humidity and triangulations, besides noting what the local people looked like whenever they met any Fort Ware Sekanis. He also took many photographs.

As we walked along this strange bush highway at Beaver Pass, it was not difficult to imagine Bedaux travelling along with his horses. Two of the half-track Citroens had been abandoned at the Halfway River on the other side of the Rockies and another two were lost over a cliff in the Rockies in a rather spectacularly filmed episode orchestrated by Bedaux. The last Citroen was let go adrift on the Halfway River but it got hung up on a sandbar and spoiled the effect that Bedaux had wanted for his film. It was difficult to imagine him with all the paraphernalia he reportedly carried into the wilderness—a silver tea service, fine linens, ladies' gowns fit for royalty, and cases of champagne, to name only a few items that he, his wife Fern, Madame Chiesa, a lady friend and their maid Josephine, all took along. Their supplies reportedly weighed twenty tonnes in all.

The adventurous Bedaux, after travelling north through country that looked as though it could have paralleled where the Alaska Highway was built many years later on the west side of the Rocky Mountains, turned west. After humbly naming a pass and a mountain after himself as he passed through, he came to the Kwadacha River, which he followed down to the Finlay River and then to Fort Ware, which is called "Whitewater" on Bedaux's map. He arrived at Sifton Pass by horseback in late September or early October, along with his retinue. He had been beleaguered with heavy rain almost every day of the expedition, and then at Sifton Pass a heavy, wet snowfall brought the expedition to a standstill. Bedaux terminated the expedition right there, and travelled south, back down the Davie Trail to Fort Ware, which took five days. In a flotilla of riverboats, he left northern British Columbia, floating down the Finlay and the Peace rivers. Only 90 of his original 130 horses made it back. It had cost him $250,000 (in pre-war dollars).

During World War II, Bedaux was supervising the construction of a German fuel pipeline for the Nazis in North Africa when he was arrested in the Sahara by the American army because of his declared German sympathies. He was taken to the United States, where he was put on trial. While waiting for the court in Miami, he committed suicide. It was May 1944.

We thought of Bedaux's luxuries when we stopped and ate a small amount of beaver meat and huckleberries for lunch, and drank water from a stream. I do believe that we were happier than the pretentious Bedaux!

Charlie supplied an interesting anecdote which I would like to think was connected to the Bedaux expedition, but could really have come from any other source. One day, Charlie was walking up the trail near Beaver Pass and decided to sit down to wait for his companions to catch up to him. As he cast his eyes around, he saw a peculiar-shaped root sticking up a few inches above the ground. Being curious and not the sort to sit around without anything to do, he walked over to the root and poked it with his foot. He then saw that it looked more like a piece of metal, so he dug around it with his heel and pulled up the very rusted remains of a revolver. The wooden handle had rotted away and the metal parts were rusted together and several rusty shells could be seen. Obviously it had been in the ground for a very long time. Charlie took it home and cleaned it up, but there was no way to find out where it had come from, but it made us wonder.

Bedaux also left more enduring evidence of his expedition into the Rocky Mountain Trench in some of the names of mountains not too far from Sifton Pass: Mount Bedaux, for himself, and Citroen Peak, perhaps in honour of his abandoned vehicles and the man who sponsored him. Perhaps coincidentally, there is a small lake named Fern Lake near Mount Bedaux, perhaps named for Bedaux's wife. And a few miles east of Sifton Pass, there is a mountain called Josefina, possibly named after Bedaux's maid, Josephine.

Old Friends and Home

We walked on an elevated part of the trail all afternoon. Our destination appeared quite close when we came to 21 Mile Hill and looked down the Fox Valley towards Fort Ware. We stopped and rested for a while, and Charlie pointed out some of the landmarks to me. We could see Prairie Mountain to the southwest, a small mountain that overshadowed the village. The mountains to the west rose over 2,300 metres. The creeks from these mountains all drained into the Fox River. Fox Pass was also to the west. Farther up the pass, a guiding outfit previously owned by Sharon and Martin Lamouroux had a small lodge.

I had flown with Lester Bower in the Beechcraft when he was asked to drop some mail for the lodge owners. He had tied two bundles of mail with bright red flagging ribbon and asked me to open my window (I was in the co-pilot's seat) when he gave the word, and then, on his command, to throw the package out the window. It sounded easy enough and I was glad to help. Because the lodge was in a pass, Lester had to bank the plane sharply to turn and then fly in low with the flaps down. Once he got his bearing, we would throw the mail out. We turned sharply and the plane exerted all the G forces on my stomach and I felt as though I was dizzy—the same feeling you get on the extreme rides at the fairground.

"I'll have to go around again," Lester said. "I've spotted the place where they are waiting!" Lester had to shout because we had taken off our headphones so that the cords did not get in the way when we heaved the mail out.

"Ready? Okay, open your window." The plane banked sharply again and I opened my window and was nearly knocked out of my seat by the blast of cold air that entered the cabin at more than gale force.

"Let 'er rip!" Lester yelled, and I thrust the package through the window where it was immediately torn from my fingers. Round we went again so Lester could see if the packages were picked up and I hastily shut the window and wiped the tears from my eyes. That was the most thrilling, arduous, exhilarating and scary mail delivery I will ever make—and gave a new meaning to the phrase "air mail."

From this point on the trail, we began to see the inroads that were being made into the territory. Hazel pointed out a cutblock to the southwest of Fort Ware. We knew of plans to extend roads north of the village, crossing from the east side of the Rocky Mountain Trench over to the west side and then turning north again. Most of the people that I had spoken to were opposed to the logging, especially after what they had seen happen to the areas that had been logged around Tsay Keh, where the village was becoming an island in the middle of numerous cutblocks.

As we sat and talked about what was happening, Charlie pointed out the predicament they were in. If they opposed logging to save the country that they grew up in, there would be no jobs and no future for the young people. On the other hand, not many of the young people wanted to go into the logging business. The Band had started a forestry company, but had to hire people from the south to run it because local people did not have the education or experience to manage the operation. Those few who did work in some aspect of the forestry industry usually had to stay in a logging camp for days on end, a fact which they resented. As usual, when we sat and tried to put the world right, we could not see an easy answer and we lapsed into silence, each of us looking very thoughtful, as usual.

We had walked eighteen kilometres when we reached 18 Mile Cabin on the Fox River. To our joy, we found that Antoine and Annie Charlie were there, along with their sons, daughter-in-law and granddaughter. The cabin stood high on the grassy riverbank where, to the west, a gap in the mountains showed where the trail to Fox Pass led. Split dry wood was stacked on the porch and a large pile of dry logs were cut and stacked a short distance away. Several old greying log outbuildings surrounded the cabin.

There were six people at Antoine's camp and they had travelled with six of their pack dogs, which were tied up at the edge of the clearing. Charlie tied up our two dogs, Bruno and Tyson, close to where we were going to camp so they wouldn't trespass on the other dogs' territory and start a fight.

We were welcomed with soup and bannock, and fresh coffee with sugar and cream. Antoine helped us to set up camp and Annie, apologizing that their cabin was too crowded to seat us all for a meal, sent over some mountain sheep meat along with fresh bannock. In moments, Hazel had the meat frying on a campfire and it wasn't long before we were enjoying the fresh fried meat as we sat around the fire on logs that we had scrounged from Antoine's woodpile. We then had some more freshly baked bannock, with butter and jam. What a feast! The dogs were not forgotten and Antoine soon fed some dog food and meat scraps to them. Like us, they probably couldn't believe their good fortune.

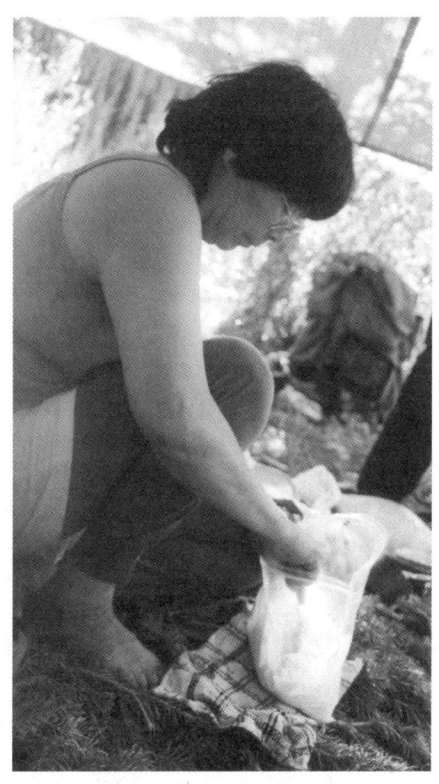

Hazel prepares bannock from the last of the flour supply.

Antoine said that they had been at this cabin for a few days. When we asked them about the note that they had left at Beaver Pass they were a little confused until they realized that they had the date wrong. Out there, did it really matter?

The rain stopped and the sky cleared, then the temperature dropped rapidly. As the evening stretched on, we huddled closer to the fire. Annie sent over some first-aid supplies for my heels that I used that evening, but I reverted to moss and duct tape the next morning. I turned in early, feeling very tired, and felt the cold seep into my tent. Bed was welcome, but after the comfort of the Fox Lake cabin all the romance of camping out was lost and I found it hard to get warm. During the night I woke up several times and pulled my sleeping bag close around my chin.

In the morning, when I saw the inside of the tent festooned with ice, I understood why I had found it difficult to get warm. I sat up and stretched, and was showered with ice crystals from the tent roof. I peered outside at the heavy fog hanging over the river and the white frost that covered everything like a thin blanket. Smoke curled lazily from Antoine's cabin chimney. The temperature was below freezing and every bit of dry clothing was required to keep warm, even huddled over the roaring fire that Charlie made. Still, I felt I could face this last day of the hike without any problems, even if I had to drag myself the whole way, because at the end of the day I would be able to soak in a tub of hot, clean water and not have to worry about setting my tent.

Annie managed to serve us hot oatmeal in the crowded cabin and I had a cup of coffee with sugar—which tasted like nectar to me—then fresh bannock with butter and jam followed. I wasn't sure I would be be able to leave this idyllic spot with its abundance of food. But thanks to Annie, we had some sugar and coffee to take us the rest of the way.

After packing—for the last time I told myself—we waved goodbye to our hosts just as the sun came up and knocked the chill out of the air. Once we were on the trail again with hot food and drink inside us, we soon warmed up.

The trail wound through a thick forest of pine and spruce trees, periodically descending to swamps of thick willows and aspen. We came to the McCook River again, where Antoine had found the easiest place to cross. He and his sons had felled large trees over the river, cutting off the branches so there was a fairly decent bridge that even the dogs could walk over with their packs on. Some of the swamps had long skinny logs placed in the wettest areas, like long stepping stones, but they were apt to roll or slip sideways when they were stood upon. The dogs didn't even try to walk on them; they just sloshed through the swamp. After slipping and sliding off the logs a few times, I followed suit. We came to several beaver dams where the surrounding land had been flooded, but we had been told by Antoine that he and his son Glen had felled some trees over most of the flooded areas, so again we were able to cross with relative ease.

Arriving at Nine Mile Cabin, the base trapping cabin that Antoine and Annie owned and where they spent the majority of their time, we found that Frankie Abou was staying there. He invited us inside for a cup of tea. While we were sitting in the cabin telling Frankie about the trail, we heard the sound of a motorized vehicle approaching. Looking outside, we saw Ruby Boya, Charlie's daughter, driving up on a quad bike. She quickly explained that she had been expecting her mother and father's return about this time, so she drove down this part of the well-used trail, which was as far as was navigable with a quad bike, hoping to meet them. After giving everyone a welcoming hug, she loaded our packs on the bike and set off for home, making our last few miles of hiking much easier.

The trail from the cabin was quite well worn, but it was dry and very pleasant to walk on. I walked as far as Seven Mile Cabin on my own, leaving Charlie and Hazel to wait for Ruby. I met her on her way back to Nine Mile to pick up her parents.

I walked into Fort Ware just after one in the afternoon, tired and dishevelled. Without having time to wash or change my clothes, I put on my business face and went just as I was to a meeting with consultants, contractors and the architect who were responsible for building a new school in the village. This meeting had been planned months before, and I had told Chief Emil McCook that I would attend it. I had walked over 460 kilometres and I was only ten minutes late for the meeting.

The people at the meeting, who had just flown in from Vancouver, didn't comment on my scruffy appearance, and I took great pains to explain that I had just come off the trail. I sat as far away as possible from them so that camp aroma might not overpower these freshly showered and city-dressed ladies and gentlemen. They were either very polite or quite understanding.

After sitting through the meeting for a couple of hours, I was finally able to excuse myself. But when I went to stand up, I found my legs and feet very reluctant to cooperate. After walking twenty-eight kilometres that morning, then sitting on a hard seat in a hot room, I think my body was resisting more movement. I gritted my teeth and walked out as though there was nothing wrong. As soon as I was out of the conference room, I limped over to the guest residence where I was going to stay, stripped off my travel-worn clothes, hastily putting them in a plastic bag, and then I spent some time wallowing in the tub, soaking my aching bones in the hot water.

Later on, as I sat on a soft sofa, watching satellite television with my feet hanging over the sofa arms so that my heels did not touch anything, there was a knock on the door and in walked Judy Sandford, the community health nurse. She had heard that I was almost crippled and had brought me some analgesics and dressings for my heels. I told her that there was nothing wrong with me that a few days' rest would not fix but she insisted on examining my heels, then she put a dressing on them. She said my ankles were swollen, so she gave me some diuretics, and I began to feel quite like a patient in hospital.

We talked about the merits of red moss and she confirmed that my heels were very clean and looked as though they had begun to granulate. I lay there and enjoyed the fuss, drinking a cup of coffee she made, and caught up on what had been happening in the village and the great big world out there.

I felt as though I had been isolated from everything for a long time, and wondered if this is what it was like for the old-timers who would have been away from contact with others for months. Life in the bush had taken on a pattern of its own, with a routine of setting and breaking camp, preparation of meals (if you had food!) and getting from point A to point B, in whatever weather the seasons or the environment cared to throw at you. We had set out to identify and visit the various historical sites on the Davie Trail and, to some degree, to participate in the rehabilitation of the Kaska Nation's Heritage Trail Project by walking the trail. Our hike was later acknowledged by the chairman of the Kaska Dena Council, Walter Carlick, who said, "You managed to accomplish many singular heritage-related challenges on behalf of our people during this trip."

We had all been adults on this trip down the Davie Trail, and I tried to imagine what it would have been like taking a family. Charlie and Hazel had taken their own family along the trail several times, using relatively modern equipment, which the Kaska and Sekani of a hundred years ago did not have. When I thought of my personal accomplishments on the Davie Trail and my present physical state, and tried to compare these things with what the Native peoples had done out of necessity, my estimation of these people of the mountains continued to rise.

Later that evening, I joined Charlie and Hazel at their house. We were inundated with people wanting to hear all the details of the journey. Charlie was in his element recounting the highlights and I endured some good-natured teasing about losing weight and having blistered heels, but everyone was having fun and as the evening went on we emptied Hazel's canisters of tea and coffee. By ten that night, we were all yawning, and despite the intake of caffeine, we were tired out. Ten o'clock was way past the bedtime we had grown used to.

"So what did you think about the Davie Trail, Keith?" Charlie asked.

Struggling to my feet, my legs aching, and then carefully putting on my clean running shoes, I took my time answering him.

"Look, Charlie, by next summer I will be as fit as a fiddle and I will have forgotten these sore feet and the bad parts of the trail, but I don't think I'll ever forget when you woke me up in Burn Cabin when you thought I was dead!" Everyone laughed and Charlie had to explain that he had been concerned about me "because I was an old white man."

"Thanks, Charlie, wait until you're my age. I'll be pushing you around in your wheelchair!" I countered. It gave me a good feeling to be able to joke around with my friends and to know that both Charlie and Hazel had looked after me on the trail.

We had hiked the trail beginning in August, as Charlie had suggested, because the mosquitoes and blackflies were not as numerous as they could be in the earlier months. We felt that we had accomplished our objective to hike the wild Aatse Davie Trail, travelling a distance of about 460 kilometres in a combined time of twenty-five days.

I doubt that Old Davie counted the days he spent on the trail. What was more important was his responsibility to arrive at a place at the appropriate season for food gathering for his small band. Travelling with my First Nations friends had given me an insight into their lives and I had learned some of their history and how they were all attached in some way to the Davie Trail that still winds through their lives. Though not many people use it in its entirety anymore, and we had only seen the evidence of animals as we barged through the bush, it is there for those whose adventurous spirit guides them to savour a touch of the past with the adventure of the present, and the trail is there in silent recognition of people like Old Davie, Charlie and Hazel Boya, and Antoine and Annie Charlie, the stalwart "People at the end of the Rocks."

Epilogue

I retired as the Fort Ware Band Manager in 2001, after serving in that position for thirteen years. I now spend my summers ocean kayaking with my wife, Muriel, and writing about our adventures.

Charlie Boya is still active, hunting, guiding and travelling to Fox Lake with his wife, Hazel. He supervises the cutting of trails and always has some project that keeps him busy although he has been diagnosed with, and is now battling, Parkinson's disease.

After a drinking session at his cabin on the Fox River, Antoine Charlie was shot and killed by his wife, Annie. It was Charlie Boya who found the mortally wounded Antoine on the trail. Annie was sent to jail in Vancouver and, after successful alcohol rehabilitation, she returned to Fort Ware where she now helps out with the Aatse Davie Rediscovery program, teaching bushcraft to young children.

Jonathan Boya lives in Prince George with the assistance of a Health Care Aide and he remains positive in his outlook, travelling the local area in summer in a handicapped-equipped van that he owns.

Tommy Poole's wife, Eva, died of cancer in 2008 and Tommy, who had a severely arthritic knee replaced in 2010, is patiently waiting for a second operation to replace his other arthritic knee. He intends to continue trapping as soon as he is mobile again.

Christie Massettoe is a healthy young lady and is progressing normally in school. Her long dark hair covers the scars on her scalp and she and her grandfather are very close.

Emil McCook retired as Chief in 2002 and is spending his retirement caring for his invalided wife, Fanny, and then in the summertime, he also enthusiastically watches over a community greenhouse project that has yielded a good crop of tomatoes and other vegetables. He also teaches senior students at the Aatse Davie School the art of building river boats.

Chief Donny Van Somer completed negotiations with BC Hydro that resulted in a multi-million-dollar settlement with added annual payments to the Band. This progressive young Chief has invested the money so that the residents of Fort Ware are already reaping the benefits with a new subdivision, new houses and village infrastructure.

Darwin Cary was severely injured in a plane crash but is now recovering back at home at Scoop Lake with his wife, Wendy, and their daughters. Darwin had been severely mauled by a grizzly bear in 1980 so he is familiar with surgery and rehabilitation.

Logging has temporarily ceased in the upper Williston area due to the economic downturn in the province but with the reopening of the mills in Mackenzie logging trucks and hog fuel trucks are once again plying the southern portion of the Williston area. The logging camp at Mesilinka has been closed and only some derelict equipment remains. The Ted Brown camp at Ingenika has disappeared completely, as has the camp at Buffalo Head (Finbow).

Aatse Davie School continues to provide a challenging and good education for the children under the leadership of principal Andreas Rohrbach, who has lived in Fort Ware for over thirteen years and encourages young adults to seek further education outside. One student has already obtained her BA in Health Sciences with the goal of obtaining her master's degree later. The teachers aides are encouraged to take teacher training with the goal of having Sekani teachers throughout the school. There is emphasis on the local language, which the Elders teach, and every year there is a "Rediscovery Program," where the children spend time in the bush learning some of the old skills of their ancestors.

The saga of the Fort Ware store continues to evolve. After so many complaints about the high food prices at the Northern Store, ownership of the store has reverted to the Band once again. It was no surprise when the new store manager turned out to be "Colins" Webster.

Further Reading

Akrigg, G.P.V. & Helen Akrigg. "Turnagain River." In *British Columbia Chronicle, 1778–1846: Adventures by Sea and Land* (Discovery Press, 1975).

Bjerky, Irene. "Cataline: Fact and Fiction." http://www.packtrail.com/faf.html

Black, Samuel. *A Journal of a Voyage from Rocky Mountain Portage in Peace River to the Sources of Finlay's Branch and to the North West Ward in Summer 1824*, edited by E.E. Rich (Hudson's Bay Record Society, 1955).

Butler, Jim. "Pilot's family to visit legendary crash site," *Whitehorse Star*, September 4, 1998.

Clare, Gerry. "People of the Rocks: The Sekani of British Columbia as Seen in the Journals of Mackenzie, Fraser, Harmon and Black." http://www.calverley.ca/Part01-FirstNations/01-033.html

Haworth, Paul. *On the Headwaters of Peace River: A Narrative of a Thousand-Mile Canoe Trip to a Little-Known Range of the Canadian Rockies* (Scribners, 1917).

Hillary, F.J. Edward. "Paper on Indian and Metis Circumstances." Unpublished.

Hoagland, Edward. *Notes from the Century Before* (Random House, 2002).

Ignace, Marianne. *Kwadacha Band Language Survey and Bella Bella Heiltsuk Language Survey* (Ph.D. diss., Simon Fraser University, 1999).

Jenness, Diamond. *The Sekani Indians of British Columbia* (Department of Mines and Resources, 1937).

"Kaska Language" (Yinka Dene Language Institute, 2006), http://www.ydli.org/langs/kaska.htm (now defunct).

Klaben, Helen, and Beth Day. *Hey, I'm Alive* (Scholastic, 1978).

Lanoue, Guy. *Brothers: The Politics of Violence among the Sekani of Northern British Columbia* (Berg Publishers, 1992), p. 168.

———. "Language loss, language gain: Cultural camouflage and social change among the Sekani of Northern British Columbia." *Language in Society* 20 (Cambridge University Press, 1991), pp. 87–115.

McConnell, R.G., and Canadian Geological Survey. *Report on a Portion of the District of Athabasca: Comprising the Country between Peace River and Athabasca River North of Lesser Slave Lake* (S.E. Dawson, 1893).

McIntosh, Deborah. "Stephen Poole." www.boothill.ca/poole.html (now defunct).

Morice, A.G. *The History of the Northern Interior of British Columbia: Formerly New Caledonia, 1660 to 1880* (John Lane, 1906).

Myers, Heather, and Aileen A. Espiritu. "Oral Histories of elders' memories of the formation of Williston Lake and its effects on the life of people in Fort Ware." March 2001.

"No one imagined the river would just disappear." *The impact of the Peace River Project on the people of Kwadacha*. February 26, 2001.

Patterson, R.M. "Introduction." In *A Journal of a Voyage from Rocky Mountain Portage in Peace River to the Sources of Finlay's Branch and to the North West Ward in Summer 1824*, by Samuel Black, lxxii-lxxiii (Hudson's Bay Record Society, 1955).

"Place Name Translations." Unpublished Kwadacha document.

Saenger, Ellen. "Leadership and Booze Don't Mix." *BC Report Magazine*, January 18, 1993.

Shelton, James Gary. *Bear Attacks: The Deadly Truth* (Pallister Publishing, 1998), pp. 80–86.

Sherwood, Jay. *Surveying Northern British Columbia: A Photojournal of Frank Swannell* (Caitlin Press, 2004).

Stonier-Newman, Lynne. *Policing a Pioneer Province: The BC Provincial Police 1858–1950* (Harbour Publishing, 1991).

Unrau, Norman. *Under These Waters: Williston Lake: Before it Was* (2001).

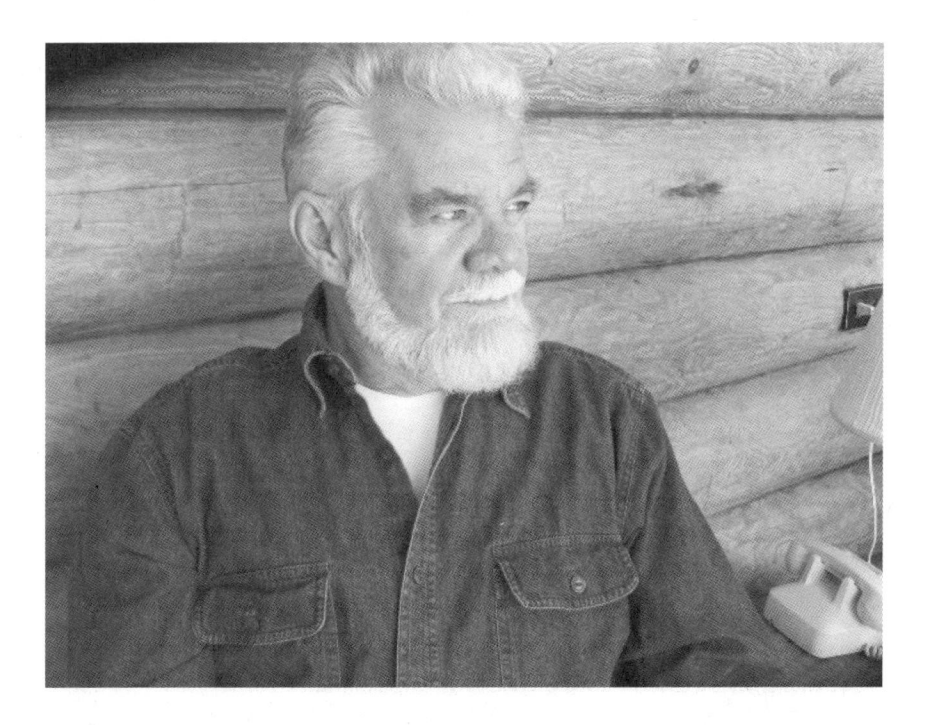

A registered nurse from England, Keith Billington immigrated to Canada and worked in the Canadian Arctic for six years with his wife, Muriel, who is a nurse-midwife. Keith obtained his Public Health Nurse Diploma at Dalhousie University in Halifax, Nova Scotia. Since retiring, Keith and his wife continue to travel in winter by snowmobile and skis, and in the summertime they find adventure in their double seagoing kayak. His previous books are *House Calls by Dogsled* (Harbour Publishing, 2008) and *Cold Land, Warm Hearts* (Harbour Publishing, 2010).